Esoteric Medicine and Practical Magic

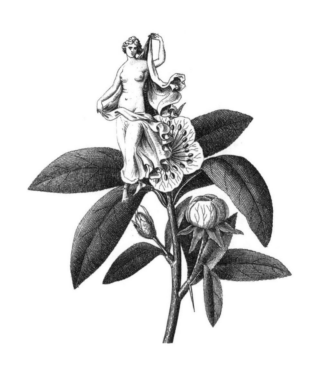

ESOTERIC MEDICINE
AND PRACTICAL MAGIC

Samael Aun Weor

GLORIAN

Esoteric Medicine and Practical Magic
Christmas Message 1977-1978
A Glorian Publishing Book

Originally published in Spanish as "Tratado de Medicina Oculta
y Magia Practica" (1952; revised 1977).

ISBN 978-1-934206-98-0

Glorian Publishing is a non-profit organization delivering to
humanity the teachings of Samael Aun Weor. All proceeds go to
further the distribution of these books. For more information,
visit gnosticteachings.org

Contents

Note from the Editors

This book has been translated from its original Spanish into English. There are several Spanish editions by various publishers, each with their own method of organization and presentation, and unfortunately they display a wide range of editorial quality; text missing in one edition could be found in another. We have attempted to consolidate the available texts and include all applicable information as written by Samael Aun Weor. This has been done in strict awareness of the warnings given by the author at the end of this book.

Much research was done in order to identify the English and scientific names of the plants listed in this book. These have been included as available. In cases where the English name of a specified plant could not be found, the Spanish name of the plant has been listed in quotations. The publisher eagerly seeks additional information regarding the English or scientific names of the as-yet-unidentified plants.

The photographs and illustrations are as accurate as we have been able to determine; however, the reader is well-advised to rely on the text as the authority rather than the images, as there remains the possibility that some photograph or another may be inaccurate.

It should be noted that some of the plants listed in this book are indigenous to specific parts of Colombia, South America, and Mexico.

The Editors

Foreword to the Reader

This book that you have in your hands, entitled *Treatise on Occult Medicine and Practical Magic*, has been delivered as a 1977-1978 Christmas Message.

This message was proofed by the author, who later added many formulae of high magic, theurgy, occult botany, thaumaturgy, elementotherapy, esoteric medicine, nahualism, etc.

In reality, we truly have written this book for those individuals who are presently weary of the many pseudo-occultist and pseudo-esoteric theories. It is written for those who want to enter into the internal worlds immediately. It is written for those who now yearn to enter into the laboratorium of Nature.

Certainly, it is very painful for us to see people wasting their time miserably.

We want practical magicians, true occultists, and not simple charlatans.

Authentic Gnostic physicians are needed, true magicians and botanists, practical people in medicine and magical matters.

The Author

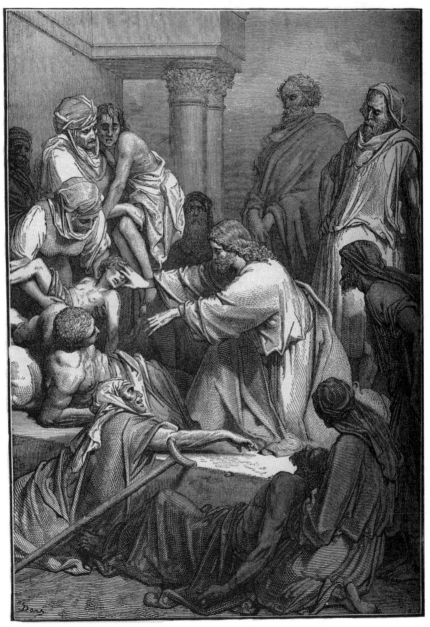

JESUS THE HEALER. ENGRAVING BY GUSTAVE DORÉ

magic: from old Persian magush, mag, magos,
"one of the members of the learned and priestly
class." Thus, genuine magic is the power of a
priest or holy person to help others.

Introduction

The hour of great decisions has arrived and there is no time to waste. We are assisting in this last moment of agony of this decayed and degenerated race.

The world has covered itself with a horrifying darkness. Painful howls escape from the cavernous abyss.

The tempest of exclusiveness has burst and the Ray of Justice is terribly shining within the august immensity of thought.

The great "Whore" (humanity) has been sentenced by the ineffable gods, and now it is falling into the fathomless Abyss.

The "Antichrist," or official science, dressed in purple, is seated on a throne of blasphemies, and as a voracious hyena is devouring human beings without pity and without rest.

The hour of great decisions has arrived. In compact and abundant lines of light and glory, the venerated heroes of wisdom are ready to fight the final battle against the false apostles of medicine.

The fanaticized forces of official science have been divided into innumerable sects that fight each other. The burial grounds that keep the sacred remnants of beloved relatives are the only mute witnesses of this quarrel.

The great "Whore" (humanity) has been fatally wounded. A breath of war escapes from the bottom of the abyss; it is an omen of disgrace. The official science of Allopathy (which was satirized from the time of Moliére until the time of Bernard Shaw) has declared itself infallible, and its false pontificates are persecuting the apostles of God...

The hour of great determinations has arrived because the innumerable medical sects—fanaticized by their exclusivistic leaders—have been engaged in a desperate and dishonorable fight to the death.

The battlefield is filled with flags. Psychiatrists, allopaths, homeopaths, botanists, naturalists, and biochemists are in combat. They repel each other on this desolate field of human Via Crucis.

Has perhaps the famous Wassermann syphilographon resolved the problem of syphilis? What specific results have the systems of Pneipp, Kilez, and Kune had on the field of medicine for this great orphan (humanity)? Has the problem of leprosy or tuberculosis been somewhat solved at least?

What happened with the experiments of Haneman and Schussler? Perchance, did these experiments cure the human beings of typhus and variola?

What about you, ingenuous botanists, who have profaned the plant kingdom by converting it into products of pharmacy? Did you achieve the decimation of the sicknesses of humanity?

Stubborn botanists, charlatans, and ignorant deceivers, how is it that you assassinate the medicinal plants in order to cure with their remains! Do you not realize that the plants are the physical bodies of the elemental creatures of Nature? Do you not understand that no plant or animal cadaver can cure? Do you believe that life can be animated by dead substances?

Do you not know, botanical researcher, that it is not the plant that cures, but it is the elemental of the plant which does so, and that each plant is the physical body of a creature of Nature?

Listen to me, until now you have done nothing but profane plants as well as animal and human cadavers! So tell me, which one of you knows how to command life? Which one of you botanists, vivisectionists of plants, knows in depth the esotericism of plants? Which one of you knows how to handle the elementals of plants?

Simply, each plant organism is the body of an elemental of Nature. Therefore, it is not the plant that cures. It is the elemental of the plant, its mantras, and the healing that is performed incessantly that cures.

Whosoever wants to officiate in the great temple of wisdom has to know how to command the elemental creatures of the plants. The one who wants to command life has to do the same thing.

The elemental of a plant furiously reacts against the herbalist who tears apart its physical body. Therefore, this wounded elemental not only does not cure, but moreover, it harms, because the vitality of the plant is psychologically altered with the anger or with the terror inflicted upon it.

The elemental of each plant has its own ritual, mantras and its hours in order to deliver itself to the doctor who knows how to command it with love and impose upon it with tenderness.

The eminent Master Paracelsus has expressed in his *Fundamento Sapientia* the following:

> "There are two types of knowledge. There is one science and one medical wisdom. The animal comprehension belongs to the animal man, but the comprehension of divine mysteries belongs to the Spirit of God within him."

While medical science is inventing certified medications that are incessantly changing as quickly as women's fashion, there is a very ancient medical wisdom that has its origin based upon the first foundations of the world and that has never changed its formulae.

Divine wisdom is preserved in sanctuaries that are far away from this false, materialistic civilization. This medical wisdom is zealously guarded by the masters of wisdom in secret places that are inaccessible to the "merchants of the temple."

This archaic medical wisdom can cure (with exact formulae) all sicknesses, even the so-called incurable ones. Leprosy, syphilis, and cancer become as insignificant as a child's game before the tremendous power of the Gnostic doctor who commands life.

"Gnosis" is the name of this ancient medical wisdom that from the dawn of creation has never changed its formulae, because these formulae are exact as the Pythagorean tablets. In these formulae, science, mysticism, and royal art are in communion within a divine union.

These formulae have their foundation in **elementotherapy**, the "royal art" of Nature that teaches us how to handle the elemental creatures of plants. These elementals were known in ancient times by such names as dryads, hamadryads, and fauns.

These plant elementals that are commanded by the Gnostic doctor are the "dussi" of Saint Augustine, the "fairies" of the Middle Ages, the "doire oigh" of the Gaels, the "grove and maidens" of the Irish, and the "anime" of the wise Gnostic brothers who are our brethren Indians from the Sierra Nevada of Santa Marta (Colombia).

The eminent Master Paracelsus gives the name of "sylvesters" to the elementals of the forests and "nymphs" to those of aquatic plants. The holy symbology of plants is found broadly exposed in the sacred books of all ancient religions. It is enough for us to remember the Tree of the Science of Good and Evil from the Garden of Eden, a tremendous symbol of the sexual force, within which is found the redemption or condemnation of the human being.

The Sephirotic tree of the Kabbalah and the Aswatta or sacred fig tree are symbols of divine wisdom. Zoroaster represented the nervous system and the liquid system of human beings by the "Haona"of the Mazdeists. Other symbols are the "Kumbum" of Tibet and the "Yggdrasil," the Pheredydes oak of the ancient Celts.

All of the ancient religions depict their founders acquiring wisdom under a tree. This is how we see the great Gautama, the Buddha Amitabha, who still lives in ancient India, achieving illumination beneath the Bodhi tree.

Christ is an exception to this rule, since Christ is the very same wisdom. He is the Solar Logos whose physical body is the Sun. Thus, Christ walks with his Sun in the same way as the human souls walk with their bodies of flesh and bones. Christ is the light of the Sun. Therefore, the light of the Sun is the light of Christ.

The light of the Sun is a christonic substance that makes the plants grow and the seeds sprout. Thus, within the compact hardness of the grain the substance of the Solar Logos remains enclosed, and it is what permits the plant to reproduce itself

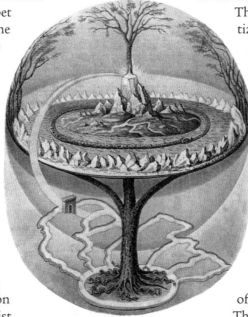

THE NORDIC TREE
YGGDRASIL

constantly with this glorious, hardy and active life.

Folklore, the history of magic and witchcraft, proven stories of witchcraft assassinations and deaths across vast distances are only possible by commanding the elemental of plants.

The miraculous healings from a distance of which the sacred books speak are performed by the Gnostic doctor by means of the elementals of plants.

This science that I baptize with the name of **elementotherapy**, the "royal art" of medical wisdom, is as ancient as the world. One cannot be a doctor without being a magician, nor can one be a magician without being a doctor.

The herbalist and the allopathic doctor are identical in the sense that they only study the physical body of living beings.

The Gnostic doctor studies the human being and the plant in their triple aspect of body, soul and spirit.

The Gnostic doctor treats plants the same way he treats human beings. The Gnostic therapeutics are mystical, symbolical and alchemical.

There are two types of angels: innocent angels and virtuous angels. The innocent angels are the elementals of plants and the virtuous angels are perfect human beings.

In the glorious India of the "Rishis," there is not a town lacking a magical tree whose "elemental genie" the population renders worship to. The Hellenic traditions sustain that each jungle has its own "genie" and each tree its "nymph."

It is not rare to see sacred trees upon the Nilgiris that have graphics on their trunks that are secret figures in vermilion and blue, and at their foot some stones painted in red.

These sacred trees are places for sacrifices and praying. Remains of animals are found there, and also locks of hair that were offered by the sick and possessed people as an action of thanksgiving to the elemental genie who cured them. The elemental genii of these trees are named "Mounispouranms" by these people.

Commonly, these trees belong to the family of the ilex. Sometimes, these trees belong to the family of the wild "cinname," and also to the family that is known by the name of "eugenie." Interesting testimonies of some wise men appear in E. Boscowits' original book. They assert what the indigenous tribes of America have known throughout millions of years, which is that the plants have soul, life, and sensibility similar to that of human beings.

In his book *Botanical Garden,* Erasmus Darwin states that the plant has a soul. We have to remember that before the false lights of this modern civilization came to appear in this world, such eminent men as Democritus, Anaxagoras, and Empedocles sustained the same thesis.

In more recent epochs, there are some who sustain that the movements of the roots are willful.

Vrolik, Hedwig, Bonnet, Ludwig, and F. Ed. Smith affirm that the plant is susceptible to diverse sensations and that it knows happiness. Finally, the sage Theodorus Fechner wrote a book entitled *Nanna Oder*

Uber Das Lenleben der Pflansen within which he sufficiently proves that plants have souls.

What moves us Gnostics into compassion is that the assertion about the souls of plants only now comes into these scientists' mind (like a very new thesis). Gnosticism has known this from the very birth of the world and it is known by any humble, simple Indian from the Sierra Nevada of Santa Marta (Colombia).

The knotweed plant is joyous and moves its branches when the wise person who knows how to love it approaches it. The garden poppy, the opium poppy, withdraws its leaves and becomes lethargic many times before being touched by the Gnostic doctor.

The elemental of the plant is joyous when we love it and it is filled with pain when we hurt it. The physical organism of the elementals of Nature is analogous to that of humans.

The respiration of the plants is performed by means of the tracheas of Malpighi that are compounded by a cellular band, coiled in a spiral, that is endowed with contraction and expansion.

According to the scientific experiments of Calandrini, Duhamel, and Papin, the only foundation for the plant's life is air. Bertholon sustained that the activity of the air in the sap of the plant is an analogous action to the one that happens in our blood.

Experiments of Ingenhus, Mohi, Garren, Hales, and Theodorous de Saussere scientifically proved that the inferior side of the leaves is filled with tiny little stomach-like mouths. These are the organs for such respiration.

The plants inhale carbonic anhydride and exhale oxygen. Their roots serve as a stomach and they emulsify the elements of the earth with their semen, by transforming them into ineffable "arcana" of the substance of God.

These "arcana" are the instruments that the elementals of plants utilize in order to heal the sick person. However, this only occurs when the Gnostic doctor has accomplished the **three indispensable requisites**, which are: love for God and the neighbor, perfect ritual, and exact diagnosis.

Elementotherapy teaches the Gnostic doctor how to command the elementals of plants. Elementotherapy is the wisdom that allows the Gnostic doctor to command life.

Until now, botanists have been maneuvering the forms, but not the very life of plants. This is because the life of the plants can only be handled by the Gnostic doctor who has studied elementotherapy.

The botanists are the vivisectionists of plants, the profane and profaners of the temple of Nature.

The allopaths only superficially know about the biomechanics of organic phenomena, but, regarding the vital foundation, they do not know anything.

The allopaths as well as the botanists are skillful in handling cadaverous forms. From the physiological or pathological point of view, we can state with propriety that the allopaths are the vivisectionists of animals and human beings.

The homeopaths, biochemists, and their kind are just the prodigal children of botany and allopathy.

The hour of great decisions has arrived and there is no time to waste. To cast out the merchants of the temple with the whip of willpower is what concerns divinized humans!

The hour in which we have to liberate ourselves from every social bondage (schools and sects, religions and dogmas) has arrived, in order to return with happiness into the temple of Nature!

We must revolutionize ourselves against every type of Theosophy, pompous Rosicrucianism, and fanatical Spiritualism. We must burn the golden calf (money), abandon the cities and return into the bosom of Nature!

When the human being returns into the bosom of his "Mother" (Nature), then she will give him bread, shelter, and wisdom. She (Nature) will give him what no leader of political trickery can give him, which are bread, shelter, and wisdom.

Now we have to return to the sublime cosmic mysticism of the Blessed Mother of the world.

The hour in which we must officiate within the temple of the Goddess Mother of the world has arrived. Thus, we will do so with the same wisdom that the human being knew in ancient "Arcadia," when he had yet to trap himself within this urban life.

We will call the archaic medical wisdom elementotherapy. This is the wisdom of the Gnostic doctors.

> "These kind of doctors (the Gnostics) are named 'Spirituals' because they can command the spirits of herbs and roots. Thus, they (the Gnostic doctors) force the spirits to give liberty to the sick people who they have put into imprisonment. Just like the judge who places a prisoner in the iron trap, this judge is the doctor of this prisoner, because having the keys of the trap, he can close and open the lock at any time that he so pleases. Hippocrates is one of those who belonged to this class of doctors." - Paracelsus, Parami-prologo III

The illustrious German Gnostic Dr. Franz Hartmann said:

> "The true doctor is not the result of scientific schools, but the one who became a doctor through the light of divine wisdom itself."

You, theologists, who know nothing about God! You, doctors, who ignore the medical science! You, anthropologists, who do not know human nature in all of its manifestations! You, lawyers, who do not have any feeling for righteousness, or for justice! You, Christians, who betray the Master in every moment! You, judges, who have never judged your own vices and defects! You, governors, who have not learned how to govern your lower passions! You, priests, who exploit the fanatical sects of the world! You, merchants, who do not have respect, not even for the "bread" that Mother Nature gives to her children! Listen, all of you, you have prostituted everything with your filthy money!

Woe to you and your children! Woe to the dwellers of the earth, because they will fall by the knife upon the sidewalks of all cities, and in the darkness of the abyss they will only hear the painful lament and the gnashing of teeth!

The official medicine has exploited human pain. When the human being separated himself from Nature in order to imprison himself within this urban life, he then fell into the hands of the tenebrous potencies. Thus, he learned the "false science" from the magicians of the darkness. It was then when he knew pain. Now, the human being has to return to the bosom of Nature in order to recuperate the lost positions.

Each elemental of Nature represents certain powers of the blessed Goddess Mother of the world. Thus, whosoever knows how to handle the powers of Nature that are enclosed within each herb, within each root and each tree, is the only one who can be a true magician and doctor.

Thought is a great force, yet everything is dual in creation. Thus, if we want to make perceptible any hidden intention, a physical instrument that serves as the clothing for that idea is necessary. This instrument is the plant that corresponds to our intention. Only the one who knows the secret of commanding the elementals of plants can be a magician.

The use of animal magnetism, the transmission of life (mumia), the transplantation of sicknesses and other analogous things that were wisely described by Paracelsus, Cornelius, Agrippa, are only possible for the Gnostic doctor who knows how to handle the elemental creatures of the plants.

The transmission of thought becomes easy when one operates through the elementals of plants. As we have already stated, everything in Nature is dual.

Those very well known systems of Marden, Atkinson, Mesmer, Paul Jagot, and the pseudo-spiritualist schools will never teach the human being the wise use of the force of thought, because force and forces are something very joined in creation.

Every mental wave has its exponent in a plant. In order for the mental waves to be crystallized, they must be revested with the esoteric powers of the plant that corresponds to it.

There is nothing in the universe that is not dual. If the athletes of concentration of thought do not know how to combine their mental waves with the powers of Nature (which are enclosed within the plants) they will then waste their time miserably.

While the human being does not return into the bosom of Nature, his thoughts as well as his life will always be totally superficial and artificial and, therefore, negative and iniquitous.

The human being must abandon his false idols and temples of urban life and return into the bosom of the blessed Goddess Mother of the world. She will give you light, wisdom, power, and glory.

The prodigal children will return into the temples of Nature when they abandon their urban life and return into the bosom of the Goddess Nature.

The temples of the Goddess Mother of the world—which are situated in the gorge of mountains and profound valleys—only await for the human being to knock at their doors in order to welcome him and to grant him love and wisdom, bread and shelter. These are the commandments of the Blessed One.

Until now, beloved disciples, you have only heard comments about oriental Tibet and of the holy masters who dwell there. Franz Hartmann comments to us about the masters of the esoteric temple of Bohemia, and Krumm-Heller (Huiracocha) comments about the temple of Monserrat in Spain and the temple of Chapultepec in Mexico.

Yet, our beloved South America also has its majestic temples, even if no one has spoken about them. These are the temples of Goddess Nature, these are the temples of the sacred mysteries of the Mayan Ray.

Until now you have only heard comments about the Asian and European masters. Many spiritualist students would like to progress internally, however they cannot because they have not found the path that belongs to them, as well as their ray and their own key note, which must be in accordance with their blood and psyche. We must not forget that in South America the blood of the American Indian predominates over everything. Thus, there are millions of human beings who belong to the Mayan Ray.

I am going to talk about the masters of the Mayan Ray; I am going to unveil for the first time the veil that hides them.

Kalusuanga - the primeval god of light, the great master of the Sun, has a storehouse of esoteric wisdom in the temple of "Buritaca," headquarters of ancient wisdom (Atlantic coast).

Kunchuvito Muya - a powerful god.

Nuestro Seyancua

Nuestro Padre Seukul

"Mama" Kaso Biscunde

"Mama" Batunare

La "Saga" Maria Pastora - a female master of wisdom.

The God Kuinmagua - This master is the god of tempests, who has power over the seasons - spring, summer, autumn, and winter.

The God Temblor - is an innocent child who makes the earth tremble, and whose name speaks for itself [temblor means "tremble" in Spanish].

These masters of the venerable White Lodge from the Mayan Ray are the silent vigilantes of Latin America.

The mountain range of the Sierra Nevada from Santa Marta (Colombia) is another powerful and very ancient Tibet.

Kalusuanga, the primeval god of light, will joyfully admit into his mysteries the souls who are thirsty for the Mayan Ray. The clue in order to enter into the temple of Kalusuanga, the Mayan Indian master, is the following:

The disciple will sit on a chair before a table. He will place his elbows on the table and will hold his head with his left hand. Meanwhile, he will perform magnetic passes by passing his right hand over his head from the forehead to the neck, with the purpose of magnetizing himself. Thus, with force, he will thrust (with the magnetic passes) his astral body outwards, towards the temple of "Buritaca," which is the headquarters of the ancient wisdom of the Mayan Ray.

The disciple will unite his willpower and imagination in vibrating harmony and will make the effort to fall asleep. While utilizing his willpower and imagination he must feel as if he was within the temple of "Buritaca" with his body of flesh and bones.

He must mentally pronounce the following mantras or magical words:

Omnis Baun Igneous

These words are pronounced in succession, prolonging the sound of the vowels until falling asleep.

After practicing for a while, the disciple will then "go out" of his physical body with his astral body, and Kalusuanga, the sublime master of the Mayan Ray, will instruct him in his mysteries and teach him the medical wisdom.

First of all, Kalusuanga tests the courage of the invoker. He appears gigantic and terrible in order to test the disciple. If the disciple is courageous, he will be instructed in the sacred science of the "Mamas."

The Gnostic doctors of the Sierra Nevada of Santa Marta cure syphilis in fifteen days. They cure the last degree of leprosy in nine precise months. They cure tuberculosis in fifteen days.

There is no sickness that the Arhuacos "Mamas" cannot cure, therefore they laugh at the science of the civilized ones of this twentieth century.

The "Mamas" affirm that in order for this modern civilization to reach the degree of their (Mayan) culture, hundreds of years would have to pass.

Upon the ice covered summits of this Sierra Nevada of Santa Marta, there lives a powerful initiate sage whose age is really indescribable. This great illuminated one is the "president Mama" of the government of the Arhuaco Indians.

This "president Mama" has powers over creation in its entirety. He is profoundly venerated by all of the Indians of the whole Sierra Nevada. In his possession is an octahedron crystal upon a tripod, which reflects the images of all people who march in order to meet this venerable elder, no matter how distant they might be.

The "Mamas" diagnose sicknesses by placing a sphere of glass over the neck of the patient. In such a way, they examine the interior of the organism better than if using x-rays. They smile with disdain at the complicated mechanisms of official medical science.

They diagnose the sickness of an ill person simply by placing the sphere of glass over the clothing of the ill one, even if the patient might be many distant miles away. Can any one of the modern scientists perform this? How interesting it would be if someone would postpone their university proficiency by making an effort to study

"Mayan medicine" in the Sierra Nevada of Santa Marta (Colombia).

"Tricksters" are the outcome of intellectualism without spirituality and these individuals have been and are the disgrace of this world.

The Indian doctors cure, and many of their healings are instantaneous because they have known about the proper managing of the elementals since very ancient times.

There are also temples of light in Taganga and Gaira (Atlantic coast of Colombia). The great initiates of the Mayan Ray dwell in all of those esoteric temples. The majestic temple of the Sierra Nevada of Santa Marta is the august sanctuary of the high initiates of "la Sierra."

Those temples are in the Jinn state, that is, within the fourth dimension. They are the great cathedrals of Nature where the great sages of the "snake" dwell.

The clue in order to travel in the astral body in the form already described is given thanks to Kalusuanga, the powerful god, child of the seven red seas and of the seven rays of the Sun.

When the disciples practice the clue they will go out of their physical bodies each time they wish to do so. Thus, they will attend the temples of the Mayan Ray in their astral bodies in order to receive instructions of medical wisdom.

The high "Mama" initiates communicate with the Mahatmas from Tibet and they know the plants of oriental India in depth.

The president of the Arhuaco Indians submerges himself into a mysterious vessel filled with a rare liquor; then when he comes out of it his physical body is already within the astral plane. In this way, in a few instants, he transports himself, with his physical body and all, to wherever he wants.

Nevertheless, these wise Indians are tremendously quiet and humble. Therefore, no "civilized" person will ever attain their secrets, unless the person has become worthy and deserves to be received as a disciple.

I have to give thanks in this book for the excellent data that Dionisito de la Cruz had the good deed of providing me with for my investigations about the Sierra Nevada. He is a resident of "Finca Tierra Grata," which is located twenty kilometers from "Fundacion."

I have to also give thanks to an Indian from the Bolivar State in Colombia for the data he provided for this book. The data was magnificent.

I also present my thanks to the Master Paracelsus, who inspected and corrected the original copy of this book, with the goal that this book will accomplish the solemn mission that has been assigned to it in the future Age of Aquarius.

I also give thanks to the Master Kalusuanga for his marvelous clue that will especially allow those Latin American disciples of aboriginal blood to put themselves in contact with the temples of mysteries of the Mayan Ray.

There are parts of the Colombian territory where aboriginal blood is extremely opulent, in the state of Bocaya for example.

The disciples whose blood is markedly "Indian" could learn to depart in their astral bodies with the clue of the Master Kalusuanga and to receive esoteric instruction in the temples of the Mayan Ray, which is the native ray of America.

I also give thanks to the Masters Morya, Kout Humi, Hippocrates and others, for their cooperation in this solemn mission that has been entrusted to me.

As well, I give thanks to my saintly Guru whose sacred name must not be uttered.

I, Samael Aun Weor, the Master of the Egyptian mysteries, am the great Avatar of Aquarius, the initiator of the new era, the Master of Strength [see illustration at right].

The hour of great decisions has arrived and there is no time to waste. We are assisting in this last moment of agony of this decayed and degenerated race.

Now is the time for us to grasp the sword of justice in order to unmask the traitors and disconcert the tyrants.

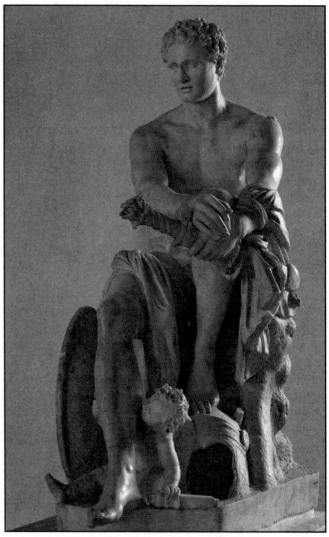

ARES, MARS, SAMAEL, WITH HIS HUMAN SOUL AT HIS FEET

It is necessary to understand the relationship between God, spirit, soul, and body. Samael Aun Weor is the bodhisattva (awakened soul) of Samael, a controversial angel in Kabbalah. Samael Aun Weor is the name of the human soul (Tiphereth; Psykhe, Manas, or the Bodhisattva), who is not the same entity as the Innermost (Chesed, the Inner Buddha, Pneuma, Atman, Abraham), or what is commonly called "God," our "Father who is in secret" (Kether, the Logos, Brahma, Dharmakaya). Samael Aun Weor repeated many times that he, the terrestrial person, was no one important, but his Inner Being is the archangel known by many names, such as Samael, Ares, Mars, etc., the Logos of the strength of Mars, that aspect of divinity that wages war against impurity and injustice. This angel is described in the book of Revelation. You can learn more about this at SamaelAunWeor.info

Introduction to Esoteric Medicine

The Faculties of Medicine

"The vanity of erudites does not come from heaven, but they learn it from one another, and upon this base they edify their church." - Paracelsus, Fundam Sap. Frangm.

In a magazine from Berlin, Bruno Noah textually states the following:

"His excellency, the rector of the University of Halle, Sir Professor Dr. Hahne states in his discourse 2-2-1934: 'I have the sufficient courage of publicly declaring myself in favor of astrology, and that it is time to recognize astrology as a science. I regret the fact of not having preoccupied myself before with astrology.'"

It is provable that the honorable body of doctors from Berlin could evaluate the authorized declaration of Dr. Hahne. Of course, this doctor is neither a "snob" opportunist nor a Galenist impostor. Astrology is a science that goes back to the time of the first ages of humanity. All of the very ancient schools of medicine drank from this fountain of inexhaustible wisdom. Since this is a fact, and certainly a true fact, the delayed recognition from this German doctor does not grant any merit to astrology. However, his recognition is with merit.

The Arhuaco Indians from the Sierra Nevada of Santa Marta, Colombia have "astrology and medicine" as the infallible, indispensable system of their medical teachings. Astrology and medicine are part of one and the same complicated organ-ism. Since they never ignored astrology, they have no need to feel regret. Hence, to use one of these two parts (astrology and medicine), or to study one of these two elements while disregarding the other, is anachronistic and anti-scientific.

Dr. Walter Krish from Stralsund states:

"Dr. Krumm-Heller founded a new theory about the organs of the senses that opens new horizons for sensorial physiology. Much has being spoken now about the sixth sense and it has been found that it has to be searched for within the fourth dimension."

The medical system of the Arhuaco Indians from the Sierra Nevada of Santa Marta is analogous to the one of the Lamas from Tibet. Thus, regarding senso-rial physiology and human anatomy, they are in an envious position in comparison with the greatly boastful ones of modern sapience.

The Arhuaco doctors study medicine for thirteen years and the minimum time for the Lama doctors from Tibet is twelve years.

The Arhuaco student of medicine remains "cloistered" for precisely thirteen years within a dwelling of two rooms. His studies are initiated when he is seven years old and he graduates when he is twenty-one years old. The nourishment of the student is administered through one window and the teachings from his instructor along with the medicinal plants are administered through another window.

The teacher who knows the least is the one who starts teaching him and the teacher who knows the most is the one who is the last. The number of instructors vary according to the educational courses that he is receiving. Each teacher has his or her own sack of plants. The study of the plants is related to their elementals and to their hidden powers. This is the ancient science of **elementotherapy**.

During the night, outside of his dwelling, the disciple is instructed by the teachers of astrology and practical magic. In order to receive this instruction, he has to develop clairvoyance or the sixth sense, which was intuited by the Dr. Krisch from Stralsund.

The procedure in order to develop clairvoyance that the Arhuaco students of medicine utilize is as follows:

The disciple stands still, contemplating upon a star from heaven, while holding a reed in his hand. Then, he strives to perceive the place that his teacher wishes him to. After a certain time of daily practice, there will truly be no place on earth, as remote as it might be, that the student will not see from the Sierra Nevada of Santa Marta.

The Indians from the state of Bolivar (Colombia) develop the sixth sense with the following procedure: At six o'clock past meridian, the aspirant places a bottle of rum, a clock, a lit candle and a plate with food on the ground underneath a tree that could be a "guasimo" (*Guazuma ulmifolia Lamarck*), olive, "totumo" (calabash tree, *Crescentia Cujete L.*) or clover bush. The aspirant consumes the food while he fixedly and penetratingly looks at the rum, candle, and clock.

These Indians always execute these practices with their face towards the setting sun and they pronounce the Christian Creed filled with faith. Thursdays and Fridays are the special days in order to perform them.

The sensorial organs of our senses are the sources of information for our mind. When these senses are more fine we have a better perception of the things that surround us. Therefore, our conceptual judgment is more exact.

The German physicist Alfred Judt sustains that a "pure blooded" individual hears eight complete octaves of the note Sol, with two lines of frequency (96.825), or with lines of frequency of 24,787,200. The measure for half-blooded Europeans is much less in their low or high auditory zone.

The pure blooded Aborigines enjoy more fine senses. If we add to them the awakening of clairvoyance, or the sixth sense located in the epiphysis gland, then a more penetrating sensorial perception and a pure source of objective information is attained. This is impossible for the students from the official faculties of medicine to obtain because of the lack of appropriate methods.

The Arhuaco Indians and the Tibetan Lamas know the human anatomy in depth. The texts of official anatomy are lacking the anatomy of the internal bodies of the human being, who is septuple in his internal constitution.

Behold, here are the seven bodies of the human being:

1. Physical body
2. Vital body
3. Astral body
4. Mental body
5. Body of willpower
6. Body of the consciousness
7. Espiritus (the Innermost)

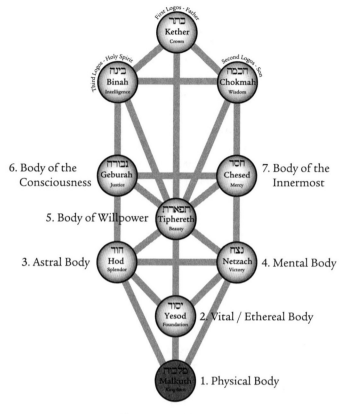

First Logos - Father
כתר
Kether
Crown

Third Logos - Holy Spirit
בינה
Binah
Intelligence

Second Logos - Son
חכמה
Chokmah
Wisdom

6. Body of the
Consciousness

גבורה
Geburah
Justice

חסד
Chesed
Mercy

7. Body of the
Innermost

5. Body of Willpower

תפארת
Tiphereth
Beauty

3. Astral Body

הוד
Hod
Splendor

נצח
Netzach
Victory

4. Mental Body

יסוד
Yesod
Foundation

2. Vital / Ethereal Body

מלכות
Malkuth
Kingdom

1. Physical Body

KABBALAH AND THE SEVEN BODIES

The illustrious Master Paracelsus classifies them as follows:

1. The Limbus
2. The Mumia
3. The Archaous
4. The Sidereal body
5. Adech (the internal man or Mental body made of the flesh of Adam)
6. Aluech
7. Body of the Innermost

These are the seven organisms made of distinct matters or degrees of subtilization, which any professor of medicine could perceive if he could develop his clairvoyance with the procedures that are given here in this book.

A study of anatomy has to embrace in its conjunction the seven bodies of the human being in all of its interrelations in order for it to be complete.

Emmanuel Kant, the great German philosopher, admits that *nisus formativus*, the Astral body, or Linga Sarira of the Theosophists, does exist.

These distinct internal bodies of the human being work over our endogenous glands and over our hormones. One cannot be a physician without knowing in depth the *nisus formativus* to which Emmanuel Kant refers.

Dr. Krisch concluded that smell, sight, hearing, and other senses of the human being function by means of electromagnetic oscillations.

Lakosky, the great Russian sage, founder of the Emanative Theory, reached the conclusion that everything radiates and that everything is energy.

It is absolutely impossible to be a physician in its whole significance without being a clairvoyant, and without having studied anatomy, biology and the pathology of all the seven bodies of the human being.

The Master Paracelsus states:

"There are two types of flesh, the flesh of Adam (the physical body) that is the terrestrial flesh, which is gross. The flesh that is not derived from Adam is of a subtle specie. It is not made from a gross matter and it can penetrate through all the walls without the necessity of doors or holes. Nonetheless, both species of flesh have their blood and bones and both also differ from the spirit."

- De Nymphis, Paracelsus

These energetic internal bodies of the human being are material organisms, which the physician must know about in depth in order to diagnose the sicknesses without any mistake, without committing any stupidity.

To know official chemistry is worthless if "esoteric chemistry" is unknown. It is worthless to know exterior biology if the "internal biology" of the seven bodies of the human being is unknown. In like manner, it is worthless to know only about exterior anatomy without knowing about "internal anatomy." In the laboratory, the theoretical study of bacteriology would be futile without a microscope.

It is absurd to study medicine without previously having developed positive clairvoyance, which permits us to see and handle the seven bodies of the human being.

The methods of diagnosis of the official science are insufficient. For this reason, the majority of patients die without knowing what their sickness was.

The Indian Jeronimo Montaño would place a crystal ball on the neck of the sick person, which allowed him to see the organism through it better than x-rays would. When it was necessary to diagnose a distant patient, it was enough for him to humidify his crystal ball with rum and to envelope it within the clothing of the sick person. Thus, in this singular manner, he knew what the sickness was and he was able to diagnose it with certainty.

On one occasion, two skeptical persons brought the hat of a dead man to the Indian Jeronimo so that he could tell them to whom the hat belonged. Thus, Jeronimo took the hat in his hands and invited the two skeptical people into his clinic. Then, with a loud voice he told them: "Behold, the owner of this hat is here." The two skeptical ones became shocked when they saw the very defunct man of the experiment seated upon a chair.

I would like to see a pupil who is in his last year of medical school diagnose someone in the presence of a "Mama" from the Sierra Nevada of Santa Marta. It would be funny, very funny...

When finalizing the studies in medicine, the Arhuaco pupil is examined by all of his teachers and in the presence of the government of Indians from the Sierra. One by one, each teacher examines him with their sack of plants. The astrologers examine him in astrology, the magicians examine him in practical magic, etc. The exam on plants is related to the esotericism of them, that is to say, with the elementotherapy, which is ignored by botanists.

The schools of medicine of the Lamas from Oriental Tibet do it in their proper way. One of their specialties is **osmotherapy**, or healing through perfumes.

We copied the following prayer from a Lama's prayer book, which is mentioned by Krumm-Heller:

> "Sublime flowers, chosen rosaries of little flowers, music and ointments of delectable fragrance, resplendent lights and the best perfumes, I bring to the victorious ones (the Buddhas) magnificent tunics and extra-fine perfumes, little sacks filled with cut aromatic burning sticks, which are equal in number to the mountains of 'Miru'

and all of the most beautiful creations, I bring to the victorious ones."

Frhr. Von Perckammer painted an illustration that is mentioned by Dr. Krumm-Heller. In this illustration appeared a Lama who is on the patio of Yungho-Kung, in the Temple of the Eternal Peace. He is portending alongside of a censer.

Perfumes are never absent within the Lama's convent of the Hundred Thousand Images of Maitreya. Dr. Rudolf Steiner affirms that the employment of perfumes for the healing of sicknesses has a very remote past and a splendid future. Leadbeater said that our sins and faults bounce back into the Astral Body and that they can be eliminated through the action of certain perfumes. Each vice has its own larvae that are attached to the Astral Body. Thus, the total healing of those vices is achieved only by the disintegration of those larvae by means of certain perfumes.

There are statues of Buddha made with perfumed sandalwood in Peking, Tibet, and in the Mongolian cloister of Erdoni Dsu. These statues remain enveloped with aromatic herbs that are utilized in order to perform distant healings. These statues are named "Dscho" (written "je") because of the abbreviation of "jebe" which means lord or master. They are also in Lhasa, the capital of Tibet.

"Tschima-Purma" is the name of certain cloth balls that are filled with aromatic herbs that Tibetans and Mongolians hang on the ceilings of their temples for healing purposes.

Krumm-Heller mentions to us in one of his books that Lama Rintschen practiced medicine in Berlin with the essences he brought from Tibet; he never bought a single drug in Berlin. As Huiracocha tells us, his mission was to care for the resident Mongolians.

The severe studies of Himalayan and Trans-Himalayan medicine include elementotherapy, osmotherapy, anatomy of the seven bodies, astrology and esoteric chemistry. Every Lama-physician is a clairvoyant. Indeed, truly, one cannot be a physician without being a clairvoyant.

Listen to this, gentlemen of official medicine. The diagnosis through percussion and auscultation and the manner in which a blind man moves and walks are analogous. To use the sense of touch in order to orient oneself in a diagnosis is absolutely unsure and puerile.

The Arhuaco and Lama physicians do not need those antiquated methods of diagnosis from official medicine for anything, since they are only good for blind men.

The Arhuaco and Lama physicians have developed the sixth sense, clairvoyance. Thus, they can see directly the causes of the sickness and its effects in the internal bodies.

There is a subterranean city in the profound Amazon jungles. Some occidental yogis dwell there. The sacred treasures of submerged Atlantis are zealously kept within this mysterious city. These sage-yogi physicians are the zealous guardians of the very ancient medical wisdom.

Another mysterious city also exists within the thick jungles of California. This city will never be discovered by the "civilized" people of this twentieth century. Here is where a surviving race from ancient Lemuria dwells. This race is the most ancient depository of the precious treasure of medical wisdom.

Likewise, in Central America there are various sanctuaries of medicine based on the "royal art" of Nature. Thus, in our world there is no scarcity of secret places where this medical wisdom is cultivated and studied. The human being knew this wisdom in former times, when he lived away from this vicious atmosphere of urban life.

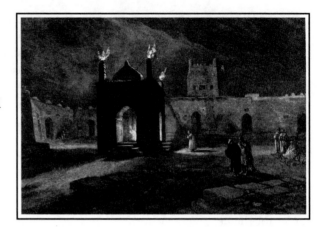

Epidemics put the world in mourning. Death advances triumphantly and devastatingly everywhere. The transitory power of allopathic medicine is abdicating before the avalanche of human pain.

The hour in order to return to Nature, the hour to withdraw into the countryside in order to learn the teachings that I give in this book has arrived.

Thus, in the profound peace of the forests is where we must establish nurseries of medical wisdom, similar to those sanctuaries in Tibet and the Sierra Nevada of Santa Marta.

Youth with genius, defenseless humanity, unsatisfied people, let us go into battle with this re-conquered flag that I raise on high towards all winds! Let us go to battle against scientific exclusivity! Let us go to war against all that is harmful and antiquated!

To the battle for Aquarius! To the battle for the new era!

Medical Clinics

"The one who can cure sicknesses is a physician. Neither the emperors, nor the popes, nor the colleges, not even the superior schools can create physicians. They can grant privileges and make a person who is not a physician appear as if he is a physician. They can grant unto this person permission to kill, but they cannot give him the power to heal. They cannot make of that person a true physician, unless that person has already been ordained by God."
 -Paracelsus

In order to be a true physician it is necessary to have wisdom. The word *wisdom* is derived from *vid, videre* (to see) and from *dom* (judgment). Thus, wisdom alludes to that which one can see with the senses of the soul and of the Innermost; to the wise judgments which must be based on the ultra-sensorial perceptions and not simply on dogmatic intellectualism or vain professional sufficiency, which are already in declination and decrepitude. Therefore, how can a person who has yet to develop his clairvoyance reach wisdom? How can a person who is not a physician to himself be a physician to others? How can a person who is not sane in his heart heal others?

Fifty percent of medical clinics (there is no sin of exaggeration here) are simulated brothels. If not, then let the other fifty percent of innocent physicians attest to this.

The aristocratic lady and the humble peasant girl adulterate within the medical clinics. The blushing of young wives or of bashful virgins cannot prevail in order to stop the outrage of those physicians who see and touch what is secret and prohibited. Indeed, they do this because of their repressed or insatiable libido (which Freud called "sexual appetite"); never before had they such an opportunity to devour women's chastity and to sacrifice their integrity!

An authentic physician must be absolutely chaste and righteous, or at least tender in his heart. Therefore, is it wisdom to work in that manner, against the moral laws? Is this culture? Is it civilization? What could this behavior be called?

When human beings endowed with superior intelligence appeared upon the earth, they allowed this supreme power (the Innermost) to work without resistance within them. Thus, they learned their first lessons from Him. All that they had to do was imitate Him, but in order to reproduce the same effects by an effort of individual will, they found themselves obliged to develop in their human constitution a creative power, the Kundalini (named Kriyashakti in esoteric terminology).

In order to be a physician, the fire of the Holy Spirit is necessary. This fire is the outcome of the transmutations of our sexual secretions by means of the snake.

How can one whose soul is stained because of love for profit and because of an insatiable thirst for fornication serve as a vehicle of expression for the Innermost?

The Innermost within us is our Internal Master, our God, our real Being, our Spirit, our superior Self, our Father who is in secret. The Innermost is an ineffable flame of the great bonfire. He is a fragment of the Absolute in our heart. According to Moses, the Innermost within us is the Ruach Elohim, who sowed the waters in the beginning of the world. The Innermost is the Monad of Carpocrates, the Daimon of Socrates, the Seity of Tibetans, the silent gandarva or celestial musician of the Hindus. The Innermost is our Father within us, the Soul is the Son, and the Holy Spirit is the sexual force, which is named Kundalini and is symbolized by the snake.

The human being becomes an authentic physician anointed by God when he develops within his human constitution the power of the fire. In this way, the divine Innermost expresses Himself through the anointed one. He then can perform astonishing healings.

A human being could theoretically study the human organism and its sicknesses. However, this does not signify that he has the power of healing, since no one can receive this power from men, but only from God.

In the sunny country of Khem, there in those foregone times of ancient Egypt, sick people were not taken into medical clinics. They were taken into the august and sacred temples where the hieratic wisdom was cultivated.

Hence, sick people came out sane and sound from the temples. A lethargy of eternities weigh upon the ancient mysteries. The delectable verb of ancient sages (who engraved their wisdom in strange embossments upon unconquered walls) seems to be perceived there in that remote distance, within the profound night of the ages. Streets had millenary sphinxes that silently contemplated thousands of pilgrims who came from distinct lands in search of health and light. Faces were tawny due to the ardent sun of happy Arabia. People came from Chaldea, Judaic merchants came from Cyclope or from Tyre, old yogis came from the sacred land of the *Vedas*...

Medicine was always sacred. Medicine was always the blessed patrimony of the Magi.

Sick people in those forgone times of ancient Egypt covered themselves with aromas within the temples, and the ineffable verb of the holy masters filled them with life.

When all of this was occuring, the great Whore (humanity) still had not begotten the Antichrist or the false science and the pontiff of all the abominations of the earth had not yet seated himself upon his seven hills.

In those fully developed ages, and under those sacred colonnades, the priest of Sais exclaimed:

> "Alas, Solon, Solon, my son! The day in which the men will laugh at our sacred hieroglyphics will come. Thus, they will say that we, the ancient people, were worshipping idols."

Medical clinics will be abolished in the Age of Aquarius. Healing sanctuaries will be opened everywhere. It will not matter if we have to tolerate with stoicism the swats from the claws of the beast, whose number is 666. To the battle, children of the light, for our ideas, for the triumph of truth and goodness, to the battle!

Healing Sanctuaries

We are in a solitary spot of a tropical forest. Here everything breathes a profound mysterious air. A long time ago, a race of illuminated sages once lived in this place, before our beloved Americas were invaded by the Spanish hordes.

In this stead named Coveñas, in the state of Bolivar close to the town of San Andres, Colombia, is where some Gnostic sages of an indigenous race still live. We are at the outlook of an enchanted well. A silvester, a creepy crawling creature called a "cienpies" (centipede) by the natives of that region walks around the well, then it disappears within the waters.

Everything is saturated by a mysterious air. Some mummies that have become petrified over the centuries seem like they are spying upon all of our actions.

We are before the presence of a healing sanctuary.

Some pilgrims who come from distant lands in search of health are muttering prayers of pity. This is the way they ask permission from the defunct Mama who heals to enter into his sanctuary where his mummy seems to smile.

It is an essential obligation for all the pilgrims to ask permission of the defunct one in order to move ahead. When the pilgrim violates this precept, then the sky fills with dense, large, black clouds and a terrible tempest is unleashed. It seems as if the indignant Mama is whipping the region with his fiery whip.

Some riches (that no one dares to touch because they are enchanted) exist in this stead.

When approaching the mummy, these pilgrims collect some plants, soil or metals, with which they are miraculously cured...

This Mama, in spite of being dead, keeps commanding and healing. Undoubtedly, he is a king and priest of the universe.

This is what a Gnostic priest is, he is a king and a priest of the universe, who knows how to command and to bless.

The healing sanctuary of every Gnostic doctor must have its altar made of cypress wood or scented wood. It is necessary to wash the wooden altar with hot water and perfumed soap before it is consecrated.

The altar-table is consecrated when it is rubbed with a sponge imbibed with rose water and when it is smeared with a mastic made from white virgin wax, evergreen resin, frankincense, aloe, thyme, pine resin, and smyrna incense.

The altar-table can also be made out of cedar wood, which is the wood of Joseph the initiate, the father of Jesus of Nazareth. Cedar has great hidden powers.

The gigantic cedars of the forests communicate amongst themselves by means of lugubrious thuds that resound in remote sites on Good Thursdays and Good Fridays.

A tablecloth must always be over the altar-table of the healing sanctuary, and over this a folded tablecloth is placed that is embroidered with pictures that represent dramas from Christ's Passion. These embroidered tablecloths are similar to the corporal of the Roman Church.

The cups and sacred chalices, as well as the vessels that are filled with vegetable substances that are given to the sick people to drink, must be placed over the embroidered tablecloth.

The phial filled with perfumes (which is a metallic cylindrical and prismatic cup, with a base or foot of a goblet) must not be missing on this altar-table either. This phial must have over its lid a little metallic tower or little metallic flag made out of tin or copper, which are the metals of Jupiter and Venus.

In order to cure the sick person, the patient must be surrounded by intense perfumes. Frankincense is the principal vehicle for the curative waves of the mind of the medic-magician, in combination with the vegetable elementals.

Some aromatic plants can be added to the frankincense such as flowers of cyprus, spikenard, saffron, amber, calamus, aloe and powder from spices.

The Gnostic medic will never use perfumes or scented substances that contain mineral substances, because those are used in order to perform black magic.

The perfumes shall be blessed with the following prayer:

> *Praise be thou, oh Lord our God, king of the world, who created all the species of aromas.*

Tibetan medicine divides the scented essences into five groups: repugnant, penetrating, piquant, aromatic, rancid, and savory.

Sick people who require curative perfumes will be medicated with the utensil for perfumes.

Perfumed candles shall never be missing upon the altar of the Gnostic medic, because the fire of the candles acts in an effective way over the subconsciousness of the sick person. In Tibet, the philosopher Mahayana wrote a whole book about the preparation of perfumed candles.

The Gnostic medic must extinguish the fire of a candle within a cup of wine after every curative operation. This is an action of thanksgiving to the gods of fire.

In every healing sanctuary, twelve balls of cloth filled with aromatic herbs must be hung from the ceiling. Each ball will contain the corresponding herbs related to the zodiacal sign. Therefore, the twelve balls will contain the herbs of the twelve zodiacal signs.

A sick person will feel an improvement in health begin when inhaling the curative perfumes of his or her zodiacal sign.

The folklorist Garay describes in his book *Traditions and Chants from Panama* how the shamans envelop the sick people with perfumes and how these shamans chant mantras to them while they are medicated.

The healing sanctuaries must have a floor of white and black tiles and the Gnostic medic must use a colored robe in his sanctum. Evil thoughts must never profane the sanctuary whose portal must have this inscription displayed:

**Thou Who Enters,
Leave Thy Evil Thoughts Behind**

Diagnostic System

Presently, there are innumerable systems of diagnosis that in depth are nothing more than simple guides for the blind. These systems guide fanatical blind people of different medical schools throughout their complex and tortuous ways of organism symptomatology.

Ninety percent of people die ignoring the cause of their sicknesses.

There are many who say that the human being is a microcosm. Yet, few are those who comprehend what this signifies.

Just as the universe is an organism with all of its constellations, likewise, the human being is a world in himself. Just as the visible firmament (space) is not governed by any creature, likewise the firmament that is within the human being (the mind) is not subjected to any other creature. This firmament (mental sphere) in the human being has its planets and stars (mental states), as well as its elevations, conjunctions and oppositions (states of being related with sentiments, thoughts, emotions, ideas, love, and hatred) and can be labeled as you wish.

Just as all the celestial bodies in space are united to one another by invisible links, so the organs within the human being are not entirely independent of one another, but they are subordinated amongst themselves by certain degrees.

> "The heart is a Sun, the brain is its Moon, the spleen is its Saturn, the liver its Jupiter, the lungs its Mercury and the kidneys its Venus." - Paramirum III, 4, Paracelsus

Esoterically, the sun of our organism is Saturn, Mercury is the chest and the "fior" are the sexual organs. The map of the stars is within the human organism. Saturn is the sun that governs the belly. For more details read our *Zodiacal Course*.

Organs, nerves, muscles, etc., are only the physical instruments of certain principles and powers in which their activity is based.

In order for one to exactly diagnose a sickness, clairvoyance is necessary. Every sickness has its causes within the interior universe of the human being. Thus, in order to enter within this profound interior universe, one needs to be clairvoyant.

Freud approached this reality with his psychoanalysis. However, he did not delve into it completely, because he lacked the development of his clairvoyance or sixth sense.

The diagnosis by percussion and auscultation is already very antiquated. Consequently, a major amount of doctors are abandoning it.

Iridology, so proclaimed by the great iridologist Vidarrauzaga, is also deficient, because the lines of the iris are so extremely fine that even with lenses that are six times magnified they can easily mislead the medic.

Medical chirology, so proclaimed by Dr. Krumm-Heller (Huiracocha), has the same defects as iridology, since the lines of the hands present signs of sicknesses very complex and very difficult to diagnose. These are confusing and untranslatable in many cases.

We bring into account the scandalous event that happened some years ago in a college of Bogota, Colombia. A commission of physicians, sickened by carnal passion, presented themselves at a college for girls in order to perform sexual examinations. It was then that the Dr. Laureano Gomez energetically protested in the name of society because of this kind of infamy.

This clearly reveals to us to what limit the sadism of these false apostles of medicine has reached. Their refined lechery does not even respect the purity of innocent girls.

The doctors from hospitals of charity have converted those institutions into centers of corruption.

The pregnant women within the maternity halls are despoiled from their dresses and in the most sadistic and criminal way their sexual organs are publicly exhibited. This is in order for those groups of bookworm-students from the university (who are filled with hidden anxieties of copulation) to study and excite their own passions before the sad spectacle of their defenseless victims.

The most horrible crimes are executed daily within the clinics with all of their instruments for surgery. A doctor who took advantage of his patients for the benefit of advertisements by exhibiting them in the supreme moment of child deliverance before strange people, had to escape from the city of Cali.

The innovative systems of diagnosis in laboratories have only achieved the increasing number of sicknesses and defunct ones. The invalids from hospitals of charity are scoffed at and humiliated as if they were not human beings, but outcasts.

These civilized "gentlemen physicians" have converted the human organism into a simple "thing" for experimentation, for an essay, for a test.

This lack of respect for the bodies of our fellowmen is rooted in the ignorance of the existence of the internal vehicles.

Newborn children are separated from their mothers at the moment of birth, with the pretext of hygiene. These "doctors" ignore that the newborn child needs the vital aura of his mother for the development of the biology of his body, which is in formation. These "scientists" ignore that when the newborn child is placed far away from the irradiation of the Vital Body of his mother, he gets sick and is in danger of dying.

To want to correct Nature is pedantry. It is unforgivable imbecility.

If we observe creation in its entirety, we will then see every mother sleeping with her newborn creature. The hen spreads her wings and covers her chicks during the night. All the animals give heat and protection to their children.

Only the deranged scientists want to correct the work of God. The mother's placenta—which should be buried in a hot place in order to avoid consequences—is often thrown into the dunghills. These "doctors" ignore the intimate bio-electromagnetic relationship that exists between the placenta and the organism of the sick woman. A placenta that is thrust into the dunghill or into the water is the cause of multiple and future sicknesses of the womb and other organs.

Therefore, when those poor mothers present themselves asking for health and medicine within the clinics, the physicians, with their false diagnosis, prescribe to them a countless amount of remedies, which instead of healing them make them even more sick.

When the Arhuaco doctors need to excite their sixth sense in order to diagnose, they drink a special medicinal decoction that puts their clairvoyant power into total activity. The formulae is as follows:

Obtain a bottle of rum, ten centigrams of internal seed of lemon verbena, one seed from inside the fruit of the sandbox tree (*Hura crepitans DC.*, "jabilla") and five sage leaves. The whole of this is left to macerate for several days. This beverage has the virtue of raising the blood towards the head in order to give force to those glands where the sixth sense is situated. We, the Gnostics, do not need this beverage. These plants can be found in the state of Magdalena, Colombia.

In the systems of diagnosis of medical wisdom, the magician uses an apparatus called a clairteleidoscope in order to clairvoyantly observe the organism. This lens is constructed in the following way: Inside of a steel tube of about twenty centimeters in length and five centimeters in diameter, two small crystal balls with stripes of blue, green, yellow, and red colors must be inserted. This lens is for clairvoyance as the microscope is for the optical nerve of the medic. This clairteleidoscope must be blessed with a branch from a pine tree and three fruits of "cadillo mono" must be hung from its sides like balls. The "cadillo mono" is a plant that grows one or two meters tall in Colombia.

The Gnostic medic will take the sick person into his healing sanctuary. Then, with his sixth sense and with the help of his clairteleidoscope, he will perform the corresponding exam of the organism. Thus, he will give an exact diagnosis.

Within this sanctuary, the young females will not need to undress their bodies. They will not entertain any passionate person. Neither will the women need to renounce their integrity in order to submit themselves to the exam of any sexually unsatisfied one, since here, only wisdom and respect will exist.

The Five Causes of Illness

The five causes of illness are the following:

1. Ens Astrale
2. Ens Veneri
3. Ens Espirituale
4. Ens Naturae
5. Ens Dei

Master Paracelsus states:

"All sicknesses have their beginning in some of the three substances: Salt, Sulphur, and Mercury; that is to say, they can have their origin in the world of matter (symbolized by the Salt), in the sphere of the soul (symbolized by the Sulphur) or in the kingdom of the mind (symbolized by the Mercury)."

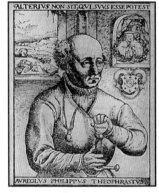

Paracelsus

In order to better comprehend this aphorism of Master Paracelsus, let the internal constitution of the human being be studied. [Read *The Perfect Matrimony* and *The Revolution of Beelzebub*].

There is no danger of harmful discordance if the body, soul and mind are in perfect harmony. Yet, if a cause of discordance originates in any of these three planes, then the disharmony is communicated to the other planes.

The Being is not the physical body, nor the Vital Body that serves as a foundation for the organism's chemistry. It is not the Sidereal Body, which is the very root of our own desires, nor is it the mind, a marvelous organism whose physical instrument is the brain. The Being is not the body of the consciousness, where all volitional, mental, or sentimental experiences are based. The Being is something much more profound.

Very rare are the human beings who have comprehended what the Being is.

The Glorian is the ray who "strikes His bell" when He comes into the physical world.

The Glorian is the Law and the incognito root of the human being.

The Glorian is the Being of the Being.

The Glorian is the Law within us.

When the human being obeys the Law (the Glorian) he cannot become sick. Therefore, sickness comes because of disobedience to the Law. When the seven bodies want to act separately as if they were seven "I's," sickness is the outcome.

The physical and vital bodies must obey the Soul. The Soul must obey the Innermost, and the Innermost must obey the Glorian. Body, Soul, and Spirit must convert themselves into a very pure and perfect universe through which the majesty of the Glorian can be expressed.

Let us look at a concrete and simple example: if we throw stones into the water, then inevitably waves will be produced. These waves are the reaction of the water against the stones. If someone casts an offensive word against us, then we feel anger. So, anger is the reaction against the offensive word, and the consequences could be indigestion or a headache or simply a loss of energies, which will be the cause of a future sickness.

If someone frustrates a plan we have projected, then we are filled with deep mental preoccupation. This preoccupation is the reaction of our Mental Body against the exterior incitement.

No one doubts that a strong mental preoccupation brings sickness to the head. Therefore, we must govern our emotions with our thought. Thought must be governed by willpower, and willpower by the consciousness.

Then, we must open up our consciousness as when a temple is opened, in order for the priest (the Innermost) to officiate at his altar, before the presence of God (the Glorian).

We must dominate our seven vehicles and cultivate serenity in order for the sublime and ineffable majesty of the Glorian to be expressed through us.

When all the acts of our daily life—even the most insignificant acts—become the living expression of the Glorian in us, we will then never be sick.

Let us now study the five causes of sickness in successive order.

Ens Astrale

Master Paracelsus states:

"The stars from heaven do not form the human being. The human being comes from two principles: the 'Ens Seminis' (the masculine sperm) and the 'Ens Virtutis' (the Innermost). Therefore, he has two natures: one Corporeal and the other Spiritual and each one of them requires its digestion (womb and nutrition).

"Just as the mother's uterus is the world that surrounds the child and also from where the fetus receives its nutrition, as well, Nature, in its proper manner, is where the terrestrial body of the human being receives its influences that act upon his organism. This is the Ens Astrale, which is something that we do not see, yet, it contains us and all that is alive and has sensation. It is what the air contains and from which all elements live. We symbolize it with 'M' (misterium)." - Paramirum Liber

Here the great Theophastrus (Paracelsus) clearly talks to us about the Astral Light of the Kabbalists, about the Azoe and Magnesia of ancient Alchemists, about the Flying Dragon of Medea, about I.N.R.I. of Christians and about the Tarot of the Bohemians.

The hour has arrived in which Biocenosis must also study the great universal agent of life, the Astral Light and its "Solve et coagula," which are represented by the Male Goat of Mendez.

The Astral Light is the basis for all sicknesses and the fountain of all life. Every sickness, every epidemic, has its astral larvae. When these larvae become coagulated in the human organism, a sickness is the outcome.

In the Temple of Alden, the masters seat their patients in an armchair that is under yellow, blue, and red lights. These three primary colors serve in order to make the larvae of a sickness visible in the Astral Body. The masters treat the organism with innumerable medications after having extracted those larvae from the astral organism of the patient.

When the Astral Body is healed, then mathematically the physical body will be healed, because before the physical atoms of an organ become sick, the "internal" atoms of the same organ are already sick. When the cause is cured, the effect is also cured.

Every sick person can write a letter to the Temple of Alden. Thus, he (she) will receive help from the Gnostic medics. The letter should be handwritten by the sick person, then it should be burned by the same person. However, prior to this, the letter should be perfumed with frankincense in the very moment before burning it.

The astral letter, or the soul of that burned letter, will go to the Temple of Alden. Hence, the masters of wisdom will read the letter and will assist the sick person.

We must have our homes clean in the physical world as well as in the Astral. Garbage deposits are always filled with infected larvae. There are odoriferous substances that burn the larvae or throw them out of our house. The "frailejon" is a Colombian plant that the Arhuaco Indians utilize in order to disinfect their homes. The disinfection can also be made with belladonna, camphor, and saffron.

Minerva, the goddess of wisdom, sterilizes the sick person's room from microbes with a certain alchemical element. This element irradiates by means of a special system that impedes the microbes from reproducing themselves. Minerva also has a concave lens that she applies to the organ of the sick person. This establishes a focus of perennial magnetism that produces the cure. We must avoid having relationships with evil people, since these people are centers of astral infection.

Ens Veneri

"If a woman leaves her husband, then she is not free from him, neither is he free from her, since when a marital union is already established, this remains for the whole of eternity." - Homunculis, Paracelsus

Really, the human personality is contained within the semen, because the semen is the astral liquid of the human being. For this reason, every sexual union is indissoluble.

The man who has sexual contact with a married woman remains in a permanent bond with part of the karma of her husband, for that reason. Fluidly, the two husbands of the woman remain connected by means of sex.

When the semen falls outside of the womb, then because of its corrupted salts certain parasites are formed. These parasites adhere to the Astral Body of the one who created them. Thus, in this way, they absorb the life of their creators.

The masturbating males engender "succubi" and the masturbating females engender "incubi." These larvae incite their creators to incessantly repeat the act of masturbation that gave them life. They have the same color as the air, therefore they cannot be seen by simple sight. An efficacious remedy in order to liberate oneself from these larvae is to carry sulphur powder inside of our shoes. The ethereal vapors of the sulphur disintegrate them.

When abandoning the physical body because of its death, the soul takes all of its conscious values. When reincarnating into a new physical body, the soul then brings all of its conscious values; they could be good as well as evil. These values are positive and negative energies. Every common and current human being has a culture of larvae in his astral atmosphere. These have such strange forms that are too odd to conceive of mentally.

Positive values bring health and joy. Negative values materialize themselves into sicknesses and bitterness. Variola is the result of hatred. Cancer is the result of fornication. Lies disfigure the human figure, thus engendering monstrous children. Egotism in its extreme produces leprosy. A person is born blind because of past cruelties. Tuberculosis is the daughter of atheism. Therefore, each human defect is venom for the organism.

Ens Espirituale

The following strange story that we are going to recount happened in a town off the Atlantic coast of Colombia, which is known by the name of Dibulla. The majority of the dwellers there are of the black race. They were living indifferently and with indolence. One day, some years ago, natives of this locality robbed from the Arhuaco Indians their forefather's sacred relics. Consequently, the "Mama" Miguel sent a commission to Dibulla with this following message: "The Mama has consulted the 'lebrillo.' Therefore, he knows that the sacred relics of our forefathers are here in this town. If you do not return them during the full moon, then the Mama will send the 'animes' and will burn down the town." This petition only caused mockery and laughter amongst the Dibullans.

Upon the arrival of the full moon, without any known cause, a bonfire exploded in the town. When the neighbors assisted in suffocating it, new bonfires exploded, especially within the houses where the stolen relics were hidden. It seemed as if the potencies of fire had confabulated themselves against that defenseless town in order to convert it to ashes. Their "curas" (Catholic priests) chanted their exorcisms in vain and the people cried bitterly. Everything was in confusion. When they lost all hope of extinguishing the fires, the Dibullans resolved to immediately return

the sacred relics to the Arhuaco Indians. Then, as if by magic, the bonfires ceased.

What were the sources that the "Mama" used in order to produce the bonfires? Undoubtedly, they were the elementals of fire who are embodied within the plants, herbs, and roots that belong to the sign of fire. This knowledge is not only ignored by modern scientists, but also by those sects that say they are the possessors of esoteric teachings...

When referring to the Ens Espirituale our expression has to be clear and our meaning precise, because the Ens Espirituale is complex in its essence and in its accidents.

When referring to the Tattvas, which are forces of the elemental creatures of vegetables, we warn that they can be utilized by black magicians in order to harm their enemies. Each vegetable is a Tattvic extract.

What is a Tattva? Much has been spoken about this matter, yet it has not been well comprehended. A Tattva is a vibration of ether. Everything comes from ether and everything returns to ether. Rama Prasat, the great Hindu philosopher, spoke about the Tattvas. However, he did not teach how to work with them, because he did not know the wisdom of the Tattvas in depth. H. P. Blavatsky wrote about the Tattvas in her book *The Secret Doctrine*. Nevertheless, she did not know the esoteric technique that refers to the practical use of the Tattvas.

The whole universe is elaborated upon with the ethereal matter "Akash" (this word is used by the Hindus). The ether disarranges itself into seven different modalities. When these modalities condense, then they give origin to all that is created.

Sound is the materialization of Akash. The sense of touch is the materialization of the Vayu Tattva. The fire and the light that we perceive through our eyes are the materialization of the Tejas Tattva. The sensation of taste is nothing more than the condensation of the Apas Tattva. The sense of smell is the materialization of the Prithvi Tattva. There are two other Tattvas that can only be handled by the magician. These are the Adi Tattva and the Samadhi Tattva.

Akash is the primary cause of all that exists. Vayu is the cause of air and of motion. Tejas is the ether of the fire that animates the flames. Prithvi is the ether of the element earth that is accumulated within the rocks. Apas is the ether of the water that enters into action before Prithvi, because before the element earth appeared, there was water.

The four elements of Nature—earth, fire, water, and air—are merely condensations of the four types of ether. These four varieties of ether are densely populated by innumerable elemental creatures of Nature.

The salamanders live within the fire (the Tejas Tattva). The ondines and nereids live within the water (the Apas Tattva). The sylphs live within the clouds (the Vayu Tattva). The gnomes and pygmies live within the earth (the Prithvi Tattva).

The physical bodies of the salamanders are the plants, herbs, and roots of the vegetables that are influenced by the signs of fire.

The physical bodies of the ondines are the elementals of the plants that are influenced by the zodiacal signs of water.

The physical bodies of the sylphs are the elementals of the plants belonging to the signs of air.

The physical bodies of the gnomes are the elementals of the plants under the influence of the zodiacal signs of earth.

Therefore, when the "Mama" Miguel burned down the town of Dibulla he utilized the Tejas Tattva. The instruments used in order to operate with this Tattva were the elementals of fire (the salamanders), which are incarnated within the plants, trees, herbs, and roots of the zodiacal signs of fire.

We can work with Apas in order to unleash the tempests or to pacify the waters by commanding the esoteric power of the plants of water.

We can unleash or calm the winds and hurricanes by commanding the elementals of air who are enclosed within the vegetables of this zodiacal sign (Vayu).

We can transmute lead into gold by commanding the esoteric power of the herbs belonging to the sign of earth (Prithvi). Yet, in order to perform this, we also need Tejas (fire).

Prehistoric traditions from the Pre-Colombian Americas asseverate to us that the Indians worked the gold as if it was soft clay. They achieved this with the elementals of plants, whose ethereal elements are the Tattvas.

The black magicians utilize the elementals of plants and the Tattvas in order to harm their neighbors from a distance.

When the astral sylphs cross through space, they agitate Vayu. Thus, Vayu moves the masses of air. This is how wind is produced.

When a magician moves the elementals of fire with his power, these elementals then act upon the Tejas Tattva by their own accord and the fire devours what this magician wants it to.

Over the sea, great battles explode between the elementals. The ondines throw the ether of their waters against the sylphs. Consequently, the sylphs return this attack by casting ethereal waves against the ondines. Then, a tempest explodes from the agitated combination of water and air. The roar of the sea and the whistling of the hurricane are the shouts of war from these elementals.

The elements of Nature are agitated when the corresponding elementals become emotional, enthusiastic or when they are intensely moved.

We become owners of the Tattvas and the powers that are enclosed within them by commanding the elementals of plants.

The Ethereal Body (the Vital Body) of the human being is constituted of the Tattvas, and we know that this body is the base upon which the organism's chemistry operates.

Nowadays, official science and its treatises of physics cannot deny that the ether penetrates all of the physical elements.

If the Ethereal Body is harmed, then mathematically the physical body is also harmed. So, by utilizing the vegetable elementals and their ethereal waves from a distance, the perverse entities can cause harm to the Ethereal Body. The consequences are very grave.

The magician-doctors of the Indian race (from the state of Bolivar, Colombia), test amongst themselves their science and power with the elemental of the "guasimo" tree (*Guazuma ulmifolia Lamarck*) in the following way: They make a circle around the "guasimo" tree, they bless it, venerate it, and beg its service, which is to attack the rival medic. After this ritual, with a new knife they lift the bark of the tree a certain amount of centimeters and then place a piece of beef (lung meat) underneath it. They then command the elemental of the tree to attack their enemy. The rival does the same by utilizing another "guasimo"

tree. Thus, in this way, a terrible fight ensues between the two elementals of these trees until one of the medics dies.

The elemental of the "guasimo" tree is a genie of fire who impetuously lunges himself against the victim. Clairvoyantly seen, this elemental uses a cape that reaches to his feet and he is endowed with great powers.

The black magicians practice certain rites with the mastic tree (naturally, I keep the secret to myself, in order not to give weapons to the evil ones). Through these rites, they achieve the harm or murder of whomever they wish from a distance. In order to heal a sick person who has been attacked by this procedure, the white magician utilizes another mastic tree. The first thing he does is to incise the figure of the sick person on its trunk. He then makes a magical circle around the tree and commands the elemental to heal the sick person. In the same measure that the incision on the tree heals, so too does the sick person feel an improvement. When the scar disappears from the trunk of the tree, then the complete healing has been fulfilled.

Two phenomena occur in the previous execution: first, transmission of life (mumia) occurs because the life of the elemental of the tree cures the sick person. Second, transplantation of sickness occurs because the sickness is transmitted into the aggressive vegetable plant and into the black magician. The black magician becomes sick in the same proportion that the patient becomes well. Many sicknesses can be cured from a distance with the procedure of the mastic tree.

There are sorcerers who take advantage of certain plants that they mix with food in order to fill the organism of their victims with deadly worms, which produce sickness and death.

Other sorcerers inject artificial gonorrhea into their victims, or they give them dangerous animal substances to drink in order to produce determined effects. The reader can inform himself in detail about all of these things in another section of this book.

The black magicians know how to inject venomous substances into the Astral Body of their victims. Thus, inevitably they become sick. The Astral Body is a material organism a little bit less dense than the physical organism. In such cases, the masters give an emetic medicine to the Astral Body of the sick person in order for him to vomit the injected substances.

The other internal bodies are also material; they too have their own particular sicknesses as well as their own medicines and their own medics. Therefore, surgical operations are not something rare in the Temple of Alden.

A serious damage in the Mental Body, when reflectively transmitted in the physical brain, produces madness.

A disconnection between the Astral Body and the Mental Body causes furious madness.

If there is no adjustment between the Astral Body and the Ethereal Body, then the idiot or the cretin is the necessary outcome.

In the Temple of Alden there is a very important laboratory of Alchemy where the great masters of medicine dwell, such as Hippocrates, Paracelsus, Galenus, Hermes, and others. This temple is in the Astral Plane, within the living innermost parts of great Nature.

The internal bodies eat, drink, assimilate, digest, and excrete in the same exact way as the physical organism does, because these are solely material bodies in a diverse degree of subtlety.

These bodies utilize the Tattvas in all sensations and reactions. The Tattvas are the fundamental base of all that exists; they can be either vehicles of love or hatred.

I regretfully have to disagree with the opinion of the Master Huiracocha about the Tattvic day-timer. In his *Tattvameter* he states that the five Tattvas successively vibrate for two hour periods, and that each Tattva vibrates for twenty-four minutes in the following way:

1. Akash

2. Vayu

3. Tejas

4. Prithvi

5. Apas

Huiracocha asseverates that this vibration of the Tattvas begins everyday at sunrise. Yet, this is in discordance with the facts and observations. Therefore, the best Tattvic day-timer is the one from Nature.

When the weather is cold, humid, rainy, and the sky is cloudy with dense, large, black clouds, this means that the cause is rooted in the Tattva of the water (Apas). When this happens, the ethereal waves of the water are submitted to a very strong cosmic vibration that generally coincides with the position of the moon.

During the hours or days of hurricanes and breezes, we can asseverate that the ethereal waves of the air (Vayu) are in agitation and vibration.

The noon sky filled with sun clearly points out that the ether of fire (Tejas) is vibrating intensely.

Dry, sultry weather elucidates for us the vibrations of Akash.

The hours filled with happiness, filled with light, are produced by Prithvi.

Therefore, the best Tattvic day-timer is the one from Nature.

When the waves of fire are agitated, then creation is inundated with light and heat.

If the aqueous ether is vibrating, then the waters are moving and everything becomes humid.

Nature becomes happy in its entirety when the ethereal waves of the element earth move and vibrate.

The summer season can be forecast in the beginning of each year. The tradition of the "Cabañuelas" is very ancient and is already forgotten and disfigured. The right procedure is as follows:

> During the night, on the first of January, collect twelve dry lumps of rocky salt. These must be separated into two groups of six. One month of the year has to be assigned to each lump of salt. Then, on the following day the lumps must be observed: the dry ones represent the number of months for summer and the humid ones represent the number of months for winter.

The black magicians as well as the white magicians equally utilize the Tattvas of Nature for their respective goals.

There are certain Tattvic extracts that the white magician takes advantage of in order to "enclose" himself. He closes his atomic atmosphere in order to defend himself from the potencies of evil. In this way, no malignant influence, magical venom, or work of witchcraft can affect or harm him.

In the state of Magdalena, Colombia, there is a tree named "tomasuco." This tree is utilized in order to "enclose" oneself. This operation is performed on Good Friday at twelve o'clock midday.

The person traces a circle around the tree, then he blesses it. He begs the elemental to "encircle" his personal atmosphere with the elemental's protective atoms, by creating a protector wall that will defend this person against tenebrous powers. Once this petition is made, the person approaches the tree walking from south to north and cuts one of the veins of the tree with a new knife. He then bathes his naked body with the life fluid of the tree. This fluid is very bitter; three cups of this liquid must be drunk. This Tattvic extract protects us from many evils. No venom or any kind of witchcraft will harm those who are "enclosed" in this way. If a venomous liquid or a venomous substance is held in the magician's hand, a nervous shock will be felt by him. The genie of this tree will spin around the white magician, in order to evade the entrance of the potencies of evil.

When at a feast, the Master Zanoni drank poisoned wine and while raising his cup, he said, "I toast thee, oh Prince, even with this cup." The poison did not cause any harm to the master. History also tells us that Rasputin drank poisoned wine in the presence of his enemies, and he laughed at them.

Ens Naturae

What wires are to electricity, nerves are to vital fluid.

The central nervous system is the throne of the Innermost (Spirit) and the grand sympathetic nervous system is the diocese of the Astral Body of the human being.

> "As the Sun sends all of its power to all the planets and lands, as well, the heart sends its Spirit through the whole body. The Moon (intelligence of the brain)

goes into the heart and returns into the brain. The fire (heat) has its origin in the (chemical) activity of the organs (the lungs), yet it penetrates the whole body. The vital liquor (vital essence) is universally distributed as it moves (circulates in the body). This effluvium contains many different effluviums and produces various types of metals (virtues and defects) in it." - Paramirum. L. 3, Paracelsus

Upon hearing these affirmations, many medics of the official science will cry out: "But where are those internal bodies?" "What do we do in order to identify and perceive them?" "We only accept what is analyzed in the laboratory and what is submitted to the studies of the systems that we have developed." In other words, the limit of their learning capacity is in relation with the apparatuses they have perfected. Therefore, the position in which they place themselves is absurd, that is to deny all that they cannot comprehend and to submit everything to the judgment of their "five senses." If they were to develop their clairvoyance, which is the "sixth sense," they then would be aware of the truth concerning this assertion.

One must not forget that the "luminaries" (intellectuals) from the epoch of Pasteur mocked him when he affirmed his famous theories, which later made him a celebrity. Did this not also occur (to a far worse degree) with Copernicus and Galileo when they became victims of what was believed to be opposed to the known or revealed truth? Was it not the "wise" ones who smeared Columbus with slanders because he announced the existence of a new world beyond the Cove of Finisterre (which was then believed to be the end of the Earth)?

The sixth sense can be awakened with the following procedure: for a period of ten minutes every day seat yourself at a table, then fixedly look at the water contained in a glass. With this daily practice, in time clairvoyance will finally awaken. The vowel "**I**" [pronounced like the vowel sound found in the word "bee"], when vocalized daily for one hour, will produce the same results. Hence, clairvoyance will awaken and the internal bodies will be seen and their anatomy can be studied.

When the Ethereal Body of the human being is weakened, then by the action of reflection the physical organism becomes sick. The Ethereal Body has its physical center in the spleen. The solar energies, which are the vital principle of everything that exists, enter through the spleen into our physical organism. The Ethereal Body is an exact duplicate of the physical body, and it is made up of Tattvas.

Each ethereal atom penetrates into each physical atom and an intense vibration is produced. All of the chemical processes of the organism are developed based on the Ethereal Body or second organism.

Every organ of the physical body becomes sick when its ethereal counterpart has become sick; when the Ethereal Body is healed the physical body is healed as well.

The disciples who cannot remember their astral experiences must submit their Ethereal Body to a surgical operation that the Nirmanakayas perform in the First Hall of Nirvana (the first subplane of Nirvana referred to in Theosophy). After this operation, the disciple can take into his astral travels the ethers that he needs in order to bring back his memories.

The Ethereal Body is composed of four ethers: Chemical Ether, Ether of Life, Luminous Ether, and Reflective Ether. The

Chemical Ether and Ether of Life serve as a source for the manifestation of the forces that work in the biochemical and physiological processes, and in all that is related to the reproduction of the races.

Light, heat, color, and sound identify themselves with the Luminous and Reflective Ethers. The Sapient Soul expresses herself within these two ethers. She is the beloved Maiden of our Memories. When seen clairvoyantly, this Maiden looks like a beautiful lady within the Ethereal Body.

It is necessary for the disciple to learn how to take the beloved Maiden of our Memories into his astral travels in order to bring the memory of all that he sees and hears within the internal worlds. She serves as a mediator between the senses of the physical brain and the ultrasensible senses of the Astral Body. It comes to be (if the concept fits) that she is like the storage space of memory.

While in bed, at the time of sleep, invoke your Innermost in the following way:

> *Father of mine, Thou who art my real Being, I beseech Thee with all of my heart and with all of my soul to take the beloved Maiden of my Memories out from my Ethereal Body, with the goal of not forgetting anything when returning into my physical body.*

Then, while becoming sleepy pronounce the mantras:

Laaaa Raaaa Ssssss

The letter "S" must have a high pitched and sharp sound, similar to that produced by air brakes. When the disciple finds himself between vigil and dreaming, then he has to get up from his bed, leave his room and travel to the Gnostic Church.

This last action must be done with confidence and faith, because it is real and not fictitious. Neither mentalism nor suggestion exist in this practice. You must get up very carefully from your bed, so as not to wake yourself. Then, you must leave your room by walking as naturally as you do when you travel daily to your job. Before leaving your room, you must perform a little jump with the intention of floating. If you float, then direct yourself towards the Gnostic Church, or to the house of the sick person whom you need to heal. Yet, if you do not float when performing the little jump, then return to your bed and repeat the experiment.

During this practice, do not worry about your physical body. Let Nature take care of it, and do not doubt, because if you do, the experiment will be lost.

The brain has a very fine tissue that is the physical vehicle for astral memories. When this tissue is damaged, the memories are unattainable; this wound can only be healed within the Temple of Alden by means of the healing powers of the masters.

The seminal canals have certain atoms that typify our past reincarnations. These atoms are also the bearers of our inheritance and illnesses that we suffered in our past lives, as well as the sicknesses suffered by our forefathers.

The germinal cell of the spermatozoid is septuple in its internal constitution, and through it we receive the biological and psychological inheritance from our parents. Our character and talent are an exclusive patrimony of the ego. Therefore, they separate themselves from the atavistic current.

There is a hospital or healing house within the heart of the Sun where opportune assistance is granted to many disincarnated initiates in order to cure their internal bodies.

The aura of an innocent child is a panacea for sick Mental Bodies. Thus, people who suffer from mental sicknesses will find great relief by sleeping close to an innocent child. Also, smudgings done with the smoke of toasted corn are very commendable.

The sick person must keep his stomach free from gases in order to avoid the ascension of them towards the brain and causing major derangement.

Castor oil is very commendable for people who are sick in their minds. This oil must be applied daily to the head.

Vaccinations must be restricted in all cases, because they damage the Astral Body of people.

If you wish to receive the help of the Masters Paracelsus, Hippocrates, Galenus, Hermes, etc., then you must write a letter to the Temple of Alden and ask for their medical attention.

The Tattvas intensely vibrate and palpitate with the impulse of the elemental populace and with the influence of the stars. The Tattvas and the elementals from the plants are the basis of esoteric medicine.

Purulent tumors in the fingers can generally be cured by alternately submerging the affected part within hot and cold water. When the action of the heat and of the cold (Tattvas Tejas and Apas) establishes organic equilibrium, then normality is re-attained.

Every human being carries an atmosphere of ancestral atoms that has its chakras in the knees. Therefore, it is in our knees where the instinct for survival is located, as well as the inheritance of race.

This is why the knees shake when we face grave danger.

Ens Dei

H. P. Blavatsky states:

"Karma is the unerring law which adjusts effect to cause, on the physical, mental, and spiritual planes of being. As no cause remains without its due effect from greatest to least, from a cosmic disturbance down to the movement of your hand, and as like produces like, Karma is that unseen and unknown law which adjusts wisely, intelligently, and equitably each effect to its cause, tracing the latter back to its producer. Though itself unknowable, its action is perceivable." - *Key to Theosophy*

Karma is paid in this physical world and also in the internal worlds. However, the Karma in this physical world, as grave as it might be, is much sweeter than its Astral equivalent.

Presently, in the "Avitchi" (Hell) of the Black Moon, there are millions of human beings who are paying terrible karmas. The mind of the magician becomes horrified when contemplating Lucifer (who is submerged within ardent fire and sulphur).

The mind of the magician becomes terrified when contemplating the famous Inquisitors from the Middle Ages, who are suffering in the fire they made others once endure, and who are exhaling the same painful woes they once made others exhale.

The soul of the magician shakes with horror when contemplating the great tyrants of "war" who suffer their terrible Karmas in the Black Moon.

There we see Hitler and Mussolini suffering the martyrdom of the fire they unleashed over defenseless cities.

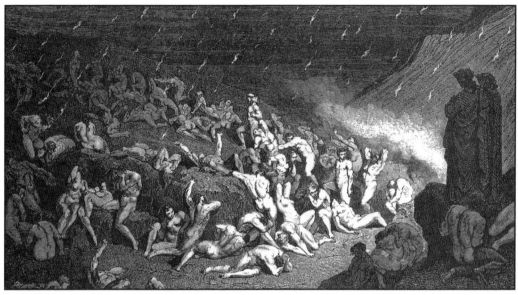

ENGRAVING BY GUSTAVE DORÉ FOR THE DIVINE COMEDY.
"The Karma in this physical world, as grave as it might
be, is much sweeter than its Astral equivalent..."

There we see Abbadon, the angel of the Abyss, who suffers in the chains and bonds with which he martyrized others.

There we see Mariela, the great female magician, embraced in the fire of her own evilness.

There we see Jahveh and Caiaphas (the supreme priest), both receiving the same torture of the cross on which they condemned the Master (Christ).

There we see the "Imperator," founder of the A.M.O.R.C. school of California, who is seized by the black magical "cord" or "rope" with which he and his followers bind their naive disciples.

When the Human Soul unites with its Innermost, then it does not have Karma to pay, because when an inferior law is transcended by a superior law, the superior law washes away the inferior law.

The worst genres of sicknesses are those engendered by Karma. Variola is the result of hatred; diphtheria is the fruit of fornication from past lives. Cancer is also the result of fornication. Tuberculosis or white pestilence is the result of atheism and materialism from past lives. Cruelty engenders blindness at birth. Rachitis is the child of materialism. Malaria comes from egotism, etc. Hundreds of other sicknesses have their origin in the evil actions from our past lives.

Within each human being lives a law, and this law is the Glorian, the source from which the Innermost emanated. The Soul is nothing but the shadow of our real Being, the Glorian.

The Glorian is a breath from the Absolute, which is profoundly unknowable to itself. The Glorian is neither spirit nor matter. It is not good, nor evil. It is not light, nor darkness. It is not coldness, nor fire. The Glorian is the law within us. It is the real and true "Being."

When the Innermost and the Soul obey the Law, which is their own Law, then the result is joy, happiness, and perfect health.

The day will arrive in which we will liberate ourselves from the universes and from the gods. This will occur when we are fused with our Glorian, which is the Law within us.

It is the quest of the soul to laboriously climb the septenary ladder of light in order to pass beyond light and darkness. The soul has to pass fifty doors in order to unite herself with the Glorian. The following is copied from a Gnostic ritual:

> Up above, in the unknown heights, there is a palace. The floor of that palace is of gold, lapis lazuli and jasper. Yet, in the middle of everything blows a breath of death. Woe to thee, oh warrior, oh fighter, if your servant succumbs, yet there are remedies and remedies.
>
> I know of those remedies, because of the yellow and the blue which surrounds thee is seen by me.
>
> To love thee is best, it is the most sublime and delectable nectar.

This fragment from a Gnostic ritual of Huiracocha (which was profaned by Israel Rojas R.) conceals great esoteric truths.

That magnificent palace of fifty doors has beautiful and sweet gardens, within which a breath of death blows. In its rooms we will be loved by our most beloved disciples, yet we also will be sold and betrayed by those same disciples. Those who applauded and admired us will abandon us. Thus, in the end we will be alone. Nevertheless, in essence, we will never truly be "alone," nor "accompanied," but in perfect plenitude.

The human being will convert himself into one law when he is united with the Law.

Genuine Powers and Inherited Powers

"Ganserbo," the great sorcerer, narrated to me how he inherited the esoteric powers of his grandmother, who was an old Spanish lady. Ganserbo said the following:

"My grandmother instructed to me how I could attend to her when she was on her death bed. She acknowledged that I was going to be the heir of her power. So, when I left my home one day, the old lady entered into a state of agony but could not die; she asked my relatives to call me. When I returned home I comprehended everything and I understood that this was the supreme moment. I then rolled my pants up to my knees in order to tolerate the terrible coldness of that deliverance of power. Alone, I entered into her habitat of death. I held my grandmother's hand, then the fire which was illuminating this dreadful abode went out. Then, a crystal glass filled with water fell and yet the water did not disperse. Finally, the old lady exhaled her last breath and left within my hand an enormous, terribly cold and stiff spider. That spider submerged itself inside the pores of my hands. This is how I inherited the power of my grandmother."

This narrative, which is as I heard it from the lips of Ganserbo the sorcerer, clearly demonstrates inherited powers. Subsequent investigations into the case of Ganserbo brought us to the conclusion that this was related with powers of black magic. The spider in question is a female black magician who has lived by adhering to the Astral Body of all the forefathers of Ganserbo. This female black magician likes to assume the horrible figure of a spider, because the Astral Body is elastic and can assume any animal figure.

Ganserbo is a great diviner and nothing can be hidden from him. Yet, in essence, he is nothing more than an unconscious medium. If it is true that he knows the secrets of all the world, this is only due to the "internal information" that he receives from that female black magician who is adhered to his Astral Body, as she was adhered to the Astral Body of his grandmother.

The Lost Word is another power that in the moment of his death the master delivers to his disciple. The Lost Word of the black magicians is written "mathrem" and they pronounce it "mazrem."

The Lost Word of the white magicians is kept hidden within the luminous and spermatic fiat of the first instant and is only known by the initiate.

No one has uttered it, no one will utter it, except the one who has incarnated it.

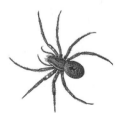

The Gnostic Church

The Gnostic Church is the authentic church of our Lord the Christ. It is the temple of initiations and it is situated within the Astral Plane. Our Lord the Christ and the holy masters officiate there.

Whosoever reads our books and practices Sexual Magic will be internally connected with this temple. The disciple can also go there with his body of flesh and bones any time he wishes to do so. This can be done by practicing the procedure that I teach in chapter five, "Humans and Lands in Jinn State."

On Fridays and Sundays, the disciple can assist the "Pretor" in order to receive the Holy Unction of bread and wine, and in order to be cured of any sicknesses. This church has 11,000 vestals. The twenty and four elders of the Apocalypse (Revelation) dwell there.

This church has esoteric instruction rooms for the disciples, in which the masters teach and instruct.

Whosoever wants to be united with his own Innermost necessarily has to pass through the nine arcades of the nine Initiations of Minor Mysteries. The aspirants of each initiation have rooms for their esoteric instruction.

Each initiation has its degrees, and each degree its ordeals. The human being is united with his Innermost in the High Initiation. This is how he is converted into a master of Major Mysteries (read my book *The Perfect Matrimony*).

The masters of the Holy Gnostic Church come to the bedside of the sick in order to heal them. There is a Gnostic prayer that every sick person must pronounce in order to ask the masters for help. Behold, the prayer:

Gnostic Prayer

Oh Thou, Solar Logos, igneous emanation, substance and consciousness of Christ, powerful life whereby everything advances, come unto me and penetrate me, enlighten me, bathe me, go through me and awaken within my Being all of those ineffable substances that are as much a part of Thee as a part of me.

Universal and cosmic force, mysterious energy, I conjure Thee, come unto me, remedy my affliction, cure me from this illness and put apart from me this suffering so I can have harmony, peace, and health.

I ask Thee in thy sacred name, which the mysteries and the Gnostic Church have taught me, so Thou can make vibrate with me all of the mysteries of this plane and superior planes, and that all of those forces together may achieve the miracle of my healing. So be it.

The Gnostic Church is especially concerned with sex.

Mistaken are all those who think that the nonsensical practices of Theosophy, the Rosicrucian Order, or Spiritism are necessary in order to be a Gnostic. Let all "Tyrians and Trojans" know that there are no abnormal people in our church. Thus, whosoever wants to be a Gnostic has to live a sane and equilibrated life.

There are decrepit old women and sexually exhausted old men who criticize us because we love sacred sex. Those fornicating elders and sanctimonious old women do not belong to the Gnostic Church, because the Gnostic Movement especially studies love, and is founded upon the sexual force, the force with which God made the universe.

Abnormal individuals are everywhere, those who boast of themselves because they have mediumistic faculties (through which are expressed certain larvae that pollute the Astral Plane). Those individuals say that they receive messages from our Lord Jesus Christ. Thus, they found lodges and societies with decrepit and ignorant old men. With their lack of respect for the most great and sublime Being who came into the world, they have reached the breaking point as impostors.

When we, the Gnostics, enter into the church of Christ, which is the Holy Gnostic Church, how difficult it is to attain the privilege of only touching the tassel of the sandals of the Master. What a difficult and laborious task it is to have the right of kissing the feet of his divine majesty, our Lord the Christ! Nevertheless, the mediums (channelers) are those who, cheated by astral larvae, say that they have communication with the Solar Logos, the Christ. What dim-witted individuals!

Let us put ourselves aside from the Spiritists and let us advance upon the theme. What is important is for a man to learn how to love, how to adore the woman, how to delight in the joy of sex without spilling the semen (without reaching the orgasm).

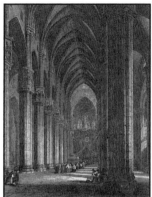

Man was made for the woman, and vice versa, the woman for the man. Male and female sexually unite, with the divine difference of not ejaculating the semen (without reaching the orgasm), by learning how to withdraw in time; this separates them from the brutish ones.

So, just as there are canals for spilling the semen, so are there canals for its transmutation, in order to upsurge it to the head in the human organism. It is necessary to learn how to use these ascending canals, to learn how to handle the snake, and to snatch the passionate beast. There is the need to exchange passion for force, for power.

Preparation and Discipline of the Gnostic Doctor

Rules for the Gnostic Medic

1. It is forbidden for the Gnostic doctor to eat any type of meat.*
2. It is totally forbidden for the Gnostic doctor to fornicate.
3. Every Gnostic doctor must be saintly.
4. Every Gnostic doctor must be clean of vices.
5. Every Gnostic doctor must be married.
6. Every Gnostic doctor is obliged to practice Sexual Magic daily in order to awaken the Kundalini.
7. Every Gnostic doctor must practice daily the exercises of esoteric meditation and vocalization.
8. The Gnostic doctor must possess infinite charity and infinite sweetness.
9. The Gnostic doctor can only practice Sexual Magic with his priestess spouse / her priest spouse.
10. The Gnostic doctor can never be adulterous.

* - Editor's Note: Samael later revised this statement when he discovered that the initiate needs to consume the Tattva Tejas, which is abundant in red meat.

Meditation

When the Gnostic doctor submerges himself into meditation, he does it because he looks for information. Meditation covers three facets:

1. **Concentration**
2. **Meditation**
3. **Adoration**

Meditation awakens the internal powers and converts the student into a magician.

Concentration means to fix the mind only on one subject matter.

Meditation means to internally reflect upon the same subject matter.

Adoration means to converse with the same subject matter or object of our concentration, to live in it, in the subject matter upon which we have fixed the mind.

The mind must be placed apart from the world, then after, it has to enter into the Buddhic consciousness in order to meditate. The mind must be fixed upon the consciousness in order to be illuminated.

When the Gnostic medic meditates, focusing upon a tree, he is searching for information from the elemental of that tree. He wants to know what this tree is for, what properties it possesses, etc.

The Gnostic medic receives information during meditation. The best hour for meditation is the one in which we feel sleepy.

The Gnostic medic will have to practice internal meditation daily. We achieve the awakening of the consciousness and the actualization of all our esoteric powers with the technique of meditation, Sexual Magic, and the power of the verb. One hour of daily vocalization is worth more than reading a thousand books of oriental theosophy.

True vocalization is intimately related with the technique of meditation.

The syllable **IN** is related with the Tattva Tejas (the principle of the fire).

The syllable **EN** is related with the cosmic mind, of which our Mental Body is only a fragment.

The syllable **ON** is related with Atman-Buddhi, the purely spiritual world, which is the homeland of the Innermost.

The syllable **UN** is related with the great universal womb, the Archaeus of the Greeks, the Astral Light of the Kabbalists, the Super Soul of Emerson (Alaya).

The syllable **AN** is related with the Tattva Vayu (the principle of movement).

The syllable **IN** makes the hypophysis and epiphysis glands vibrate. Thus, the sixth sense called clairvoyance is acquired.

The syllable **EN** makes the thyroid gland and the atoms of the Mental Body vibrate. Thus, the human being acquires the esoteric ear and the clairvoyance of the Mental Body.

The syllable **ON** makes our Buddhic, mystical, or intuitive Buddhic consciousness vibrate.

We all have longings for liberation. We all possess that longing that in the far east is called "Bodhimanda," the fundamental base of knowing. Every "Purusha" (Innermost) yearns for his soul to follow the path of liberation, or "Dharma." The doctrine of the heart is Buddha, the Christic consciousness.

The vehicle of the Christic consciousness has its chakra in the heart. So, when internally vocalizing the syllable **ON** and meditating on its profound significance, the awakening of the mystical consciousness is produced. Then, independent from the physical body, the soul acquires the power of functioning in her superior vehicles.

The awakening of the consciousness, or Buddha, expresses itself as the Eye of Dangma, the intuition that allows us "to know" without the necessity of reasoning.

The syllable **ON** also makes the testicles hormones vibrate, thus transmuting the semen into Christic energy. This clearly shows that the awakening of the consciousness, Buddha, can only be achieved by practicing Sexual Magic, by internally vocalizing and becoming skillful in the Astral, since the consciousness, Buddha, is enclosed within our own Chrestos.

The Astral Body is the mediator between the soul and the Innermost. Thus, it is only in this astral mediator region where our Monad can be liberated. Here is where all of the Initiations are verified.

Buddha, the mystical consciousness, has to express itself through our Astral Body in order to perform "the Truth," which is Buddhi, and which is truly the Innermost or Atman within us.

This mystical consciousness, Buddha, cannot express itself through the physical body or Stulla Sarira, but only through the Astral Body, because the Astral Body is the mediator between the mystical consciousness and the physical body.

When the human being spills the semen (reaches the orgasm), he loses millions of solar atoms that are then replaced by millions of demonic atoms from the very infernos of the human being. This produces a tenebrous obscurity within the Astral Body.

When the human being accomplishes the following formula, which is to introduce the virile member into the feminine vagina, and to withdraw without spilling the semen (without reaching the orgasm), then the solar atoms multiply in an extraordinary manner and return into the Astral Body. Hence, they fill the Astral Body with light and solar fire. Only in this way can the Buddha, the Christic consciousness, express itself through the Astral Body. Finally, the soul and the Innermost become united forever, thus bringing about the final liberation.

The human being becomes clairvoyant by meditating on the syllable **IN**, and on the great universal fire.

The human being acquires mental clairvoyance and the esoteric ear by meditating on the syllable **EN**, and the universal mind.

The awakening of the consciousness and the development of intuition are acquired by meditating daily upon our Innermost and on the syllable **ON**, and by practicing Sexual Magic daily.

The power of telepathy is acquired by meditating on the syllable **UN**, and the solar plexus.

The power to remember our past lives is acquired by meditating on the syllable **AN**, and on the birth and death of vegetables and of all things.

The clue of pranava, or the science of mantras, is found within the consciousness. The waves of the consciousness nourish the mind. The mantras must be felt, since all of their powers reside within the superlative functions of the consciousness. Therefore, before vocalizing the mantras we must live them within the mystical consciousness.

IN, **EN**, **ON**, **UN**, **AN** must be vocalized daily for one hour, like this:

IiiiiiiiiiiiiiiiiinNnnnnnnnnnnnn (pronounce the "I" as in bee)

Eeeeeeeeee Nnnnnnnnn (pronounce the "E" as in end)

Ooooooooo Nnnnnnn

Uuuuuuuuu Nnnnnnnnnn

Aaaaaaaaaa Nnnnnnnn (the "A" is pronounced as in far)

The five vowels I, E, O, U, A make the chakras, discs, or magnetic wheels of our Astral Body vibrate. Thus, with the vibration, the Tattvas are transmuted into hormones, since each chakra is a regulator of our endocrine glands. These glands are truly biogenetic laboratories, whose mission is to transmute the Tattvas into hormones.

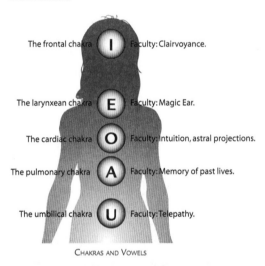

The frontal chakra — **I** — Faculty: Clairvoyance.

The larynxean chakra — **E** — Faculty: Magic Ear.

The cardiac chakra — **O** — Faculty: Intuition, astral projections.

The pulmonary chakra — **A** — Faculty: Memory of past lives.

The umbilical chakra — **U** — Faculty: Telepathy.

CHAKRAS AND VOWELS

The waves of the consciousness bring together all of the connected and harmonious thoughts in order to fortify them.

Everything exists by **AUM**, everything lives by **AUM**, and everything comes into existence by **AUM**. Yet, in the beginning, only the divine Chaos existed.

The vowel "A" is the prime matter of the Great Work; it is the Tattva of everything that comes into existence.

The vowel "U" is the mystical consciousness, or the collective mystical consciousness.

The vowel "M" (the M in esotericism is also a vowel) is the incessant transformation and existence that the gods create with their mind.

Let us clarify this in order to have greater comprehension:

The Earth in its nebulous state was "A." Then, in its processes of gestation or formation directed by the cosmic consciousness it was "U." Finally, when populated by all types of living beings it was "M."

The embryonic germ in its first days within the maternal womb is "A." The fetus while in gestation is "U." The very welcomed child coming into existence is "M." "AUM" is lived by the animal; "AUM" is lived by the human being.

AUM is esoterically pronounced *AUM* (as described below). The power of all the Tattvas is enclosed within this mantra. The Kabbalistic number of AUM is 666, and not the number ten as the black magician Cherenzi taught.

In order for AUM to completely manifest itself through us, we have to prepare all of our seven vehicles. AUM contains the seven notes of the musical scale, which correspond to the seven cosmic planes and to our seven bodies. The seven words of Calvary (pronounced by Jesus) give us power over the seven cosmic planes.

In order for the mystical consciousness, Buddha, to express itself as intuition through us, we have to prepare our seven bodies by means of Sexual Magic.

Before Self-realizing the mantra "AUM," we have to live the mantra **I.A.O.** Sexual Magic is **I.A.O.** The Kundalini is **I.A.O.**

The formula in order to awaken the Kundalini lies exclusively in the sexual act: **To introduce the virile member into the feminine vagina and withdraw without spilling the semen (without reaching the**

orgasm). This is our axiomatic prescription for all Gnostic students. During these sexual trances the mantra I.A.O. must be vocalized, then meditation on the fire and on the Innermost must be performed.

AUM is pronounced by opening the mouth very well with the vowel *aaaaaaa,* rounding it with the *uuuuuuuu* and closing it with the *mmmmmmmm.*

The Gnostic medic needs to submit himself to these rules for the wise exercise of holy Gnostic medicine. The Gnostic medic must be a magician in order to command the elementals of vegetables.

The Kundalini

Kundalini is the fire of the Holy Spirit. Kundalini is a liquid fire of a purely spiritual nature. Kundalini is the igneous serpent of our magical powers. Kundalini is found enclosed within a membranous pouch that is nourished by the rays of the Sun and of the Moon. This membranous pouch is found concentrated within the coccygeal bone.

The fire of the Holy Spirit and the Kundalini are the same. The difference between the Kundalini and the Holy Spirit is just a circumstance of names. In the East, the sexual force is called Kundalini, and in the West it is called the Holy Spirit. Yet, it is the same sexual fire, enclosed within the membranous pouch in the coccyx. The secret in order to awaken the Kundalini (the fire of the Holy Spirit) lies in the following prescription:

Introduce the virile member into the feminine vagina, then withdraw without spilling the semen (without reaching the orgasm).

This is what is called Sexual Magic, and it is mandatory for the Gnostic medic to practice Sexual Magic daily in order to transmute his semen into divine energy. Thus, the fire of the Holy Spirit or Kundalini awakens with this prescription, because this fire rips open the membranous pouch in which it is enclosed. Then, it ascends upwards through a canal situated within the spinal medulla. In the east, this canal is called Shushumna. That canal remains closed in ordinary people. However, the seminal vapors open it and expose it, so that the Kundalini can enter

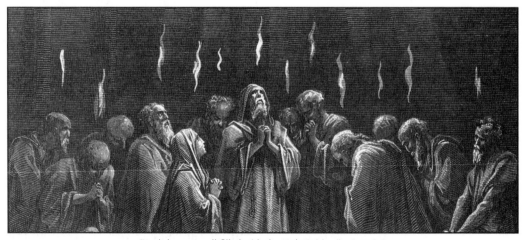

"And they were all filled with the Holy Spirit..." - Acts 2:4

through its inferior orifice, in order to ascend upwards through a thread situated in the center of this canal.

The opening of the orifice of this canal of Shushumna is performed under the direction of an angelic atom, which is situated in the semen. This fine thread through which the Kundalini ascends is very delicate. If the Gnostic medic does not withdraw himself before the orgasm, if he indeed arrives at the spilling of the semen, then this thread is ripped. It becomes a burned fuse or burned wire, and the Kundalini descends one or more canyons (vertebrae) according to the magnitude of the fault.

In Gnosticism, we call the spinal vertebrae canyons or pyramids. Each canyon is related with certain esoteric powers. There are 33 spinal canyons. When the Kundalini fire has already risen through the 33 canyons, then within the Astral Plane, the Staff of the Patriarchs is delivered to the Gnostic. High Initiation is received when the Staff of the Patriarchs has been received.

High Initiation is the fusion of the Spiritual Soul with the Innermost.

The Spiritual Soul is the Buddhic or Intuitive body. When the Buddhic Body is fused with the Innermost, then a new Heavenly Man, a new master is born.

This new master has to take out his psychic extracts, which are enclosed within his Vital, Astral, Mental, and Causal bodies. This task is really very difficult, and this is performed by means of the fire of the Kundalini.

The first psychic extract that has to be patiently drawn out is the ethereal extract. That extract is called **Arronsa**.

The master has to awaken the Kundalini in his Ethereal Body (Vital Body), just as he did in his physical body. Once the master has patiently made his Kundalini rise upwards through the spinal column of his Ethereal Body, then this master achieves the removal of his psychic extract that is enclosed within his Ethereal Body.

Next, that extract is assimilated within his Buddhic Body or Spiritual Soul. This is how the master acquires the power over the Tattvas, which will allow him to govern the four elements of Nature.

The very difficult labor of awakening the Kundalini in the Ethereal Body and making it rise upwards, canyon after canyon, just as it was done in the physical body, is performed under the direction of a "specialist."

Arronsa is the name of the psychic extract of the Ethereal Body. Therefore, **Arronsa** is the mantra the new master must vocalize in order to awaken his Kundalini, and to make it rise upwards through the spinal column of his Ethereal Body.

Arronsa can only be pronounced by the masters, yet I have written it in this book in order for it to be a guide to the new masters who with my teachings will be born.

Once the ethereal extract is liberated, the master has to perform analogous labors with the Astral, Mental, and Causal bodies in a successive order. All of these psychic extracts must be assimilated by the internal master, in order for him to become Self-realized in depth and to have the complete right to enter into Nirvana.

Then, when reaching this degree, the master is an omnipotent god, a majesty of fire, a sovereign of creation in its entirety. This is the science of the serpent.

The Buddhic Body

The Buddhic Body is the Diamond Soul of the Innermost. The Buddhic Body is the superlative and ennobling consciousness of our Being.

The Buddhic Body is the Spiritual Soul of the Being. Thus, when the Innermost is fused with his Spiritual Soul, the Heavenly Man, the master, is born.

The Buddhic Body or Spiritual Soul has his diocese within the heart. Thus, the Heart Temple is the diocese of what is most dignified and decent within our Being.

The fires of the heart control the Kundalini. The Kundalini (the fire of the Holy Spirit) rises under the control of the fires of the heart. The ascent of the Kundalini depends upon the merits of the heart. The path of the heart is the path of the Innermost. Therefore, the path of the heart opens up for us only with sanctity.

We receive the cross of the Initiation within the Heart Temple. We live the Golgotha within the Heart Temple. The infinite universe is a system of hearts. Therefore, the path of sanctity is the path of the heart.

The Diamond Soul or Buddhic Body must receive the five stigmata and be totally christified in order to fuse itself with the Innermost.

The Gnostic medic must follow the path of sanctity in order to Self-realize himself in depth.

The Path of Initiation

1. There are eight Initiations of Major Mysteries and nine Initiations of Minor Mysteries.

2. To reach the great Initiations of Major Mysteries is impossible without having passed through the nine Initiations of Minor Mysteries.

3. I am very deeply sorry that certain spiritualist societies do not know how to interpret the maximum sacrifice of the martyr of Golgotha.

4. Samael Aun Weor, Master of the venerable White Lodge, is indeed very sorry that the students of certain secret societies never talk about the nine Initiations of Minor Mysteries.

5. I declare that when arriving at the degree of Aseka, or Hierophant of the Fifth Initiation of Major Mysteries, the following seven paths are opened before the master:

    a) To continue with humanity, working for humanity.

    b) To continue within the internal planes as Nirmanakaya, working for humanity.

    c) To join the evolution of the angels or devas.

d) To form part of the government of the Logos.

e) To prepare the work of the future Ethereal Age of the Earth.

f) To enter into the ineffable joy of Nirvana.

g) To perform superior works of Nirvana.

Samael Aun Weor declares that he was the first human being in the world to publicly deliver to humanity the secrets of Initiation. If the reader of this book wants to enter onto the path of Initiation right now, then let him study and totally live my two books entitled *The Perfect Matrimony* and *The Revolution of Beelzebub*. All of the secrets of the Initiation are found in these two books.

The Seven Serpents

We have seven bodies and seven serpents. Each one of our seven bodies has its own medulla and its own serpent. These seven serpents are the seven degrees of the power of the fire, two groups of three plus the sublime coronation of the seventh serpent that joins us with the One, with the Law, with the Father.

These are the seven portals and the seven great Initiations of Major Mysteries (read *Zodiacal Course* by the same author).

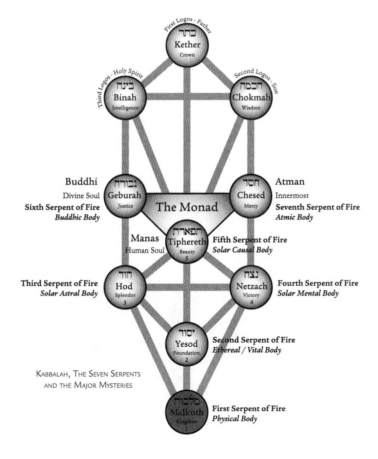

KABBALAH, THE SEVEN SERPENTS AND THE MAJOR MYSTERIES

The Choanes

The Choanes are seven, and they work under the influence of the seven planetary rays in our terrestrial evolution. Let us know them:

The Mahachohan, the divine hierarch, directs the works of the White Lodge. All the archives of terrestrial evolution are in his power.

The Manu is another divine being who has to form new races. There are various manus. When a manu lays the foundation of a new race and ends his work, then he receives the Eighth Initiation of Major Mysteries with the degree of Buddha Pratyeka, which signifies Solitary Buddha. Then, after his Eighth Major Initiation, much later on, he achieves the degree of "Lord of the World."

The Eighth Initiation of Major Mysteries is granted in the most divine planes of consciousness. The fact that I have previously spoken of five Initiations of Major Mysteries and now I come to speak of nine will appear contradictory to many people. Therefore, I must clarify myself: we fulfill our human evolution with the five Initiations of Major Mysteries. The remaining three Initiations and the degree of "Lord of the World" are of a "Superhuman" nature.

Now, beloved reader, do you want to know the formula in order to convert yourself into a god?

This is the formula: **"Introduce the virile member into the feminine vagina, then withdraw without spilling the semen (without reaching the orgasm)."** This is the clue in order for you to convert yourself into a god. Yet, to become a perfect saint is an indispensable requirement for you.

I.A.O. is the mantra that must be vocalized during the daily trance of Sexual Magic, like so:

Iiiiiiiiiiiiiiiiiiiiiiiiiiiiiiiiiiiiiiiiiii
Aaaaaaaaaaaaaaaaaaaaaaa
Ooooooooooooooooooooooo

Second Guardian

We have said that the mind lives constantly reacting against the impact of the exterior world. On previous pages we have explained that these reactions of the mind depart from the center, out to the periphery.

The mental center from where these reactions of understanding depart is a terribly demonic mental creature. This creature is the Guardian of the Threshold of the Mental Body. This mental Guardian enslaves the mind of all human beings. All of those reactions of hatred, rage, violence, egotism, etc. emerge from him.

The arhat must despoil himself of this horrible Guardian in order to convert his mind-matter into Christ Mind. This labor is performed by means of fire.

When the igneous serpent of the Mental Body reaches the spinal vertebra that corresponds to the igneous wings, then the arhat must courageously confront this tenebrous creature and defeat it in a terrible fight, hand to hand.

Thus, after that instant, the mind of the arhat only obeys the direct commands of the Innermost.

Another life similar to the present one is lived within the world of the mind. Therefore, it is not strange that in the world of the mind the competent investigators find humanity dedicated to similar labors as to those of the physical world.

The black magicians from the world of the mind are terribly dangerous... The arhat has to courageously confront them and defeat them with the sharp edge of his sword.

The Guardian of the Threshold of the mind is the second Guardian who crosses us on our path.

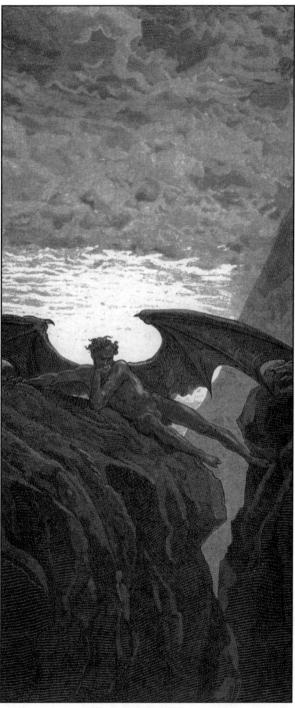

ENGRAVING BY GUSTAVE DORÉ.

Theurgy

Baths with Plants to Prepare the Body for Magic

The first thing that the magician must do in order to put practical magic into effect is to transcend his body. The body of a magician has a vibratory tonality that is totally different from that of the ordinary human being.

In ancient times, all the powers of the goddess of Nature were totally expressing themselves through the chakras of the human organism. Hence, the human being was a complete magician.

In this day and age, humanity has totally separated itself from Nature and has accommodated itself to an artificial life. Therefore, the human body now does not reflect the powers of Nature.

It does not matter if a musician is very ingenious. If his instrument is unsatisfactory or defective, then he will not execute his composition with success. Yet, if he tunes and corrects the instrument, then he will perform with it the most beautiful melodies. A similar case occurs with the human body that is unsatisfactory. Therefore, in order for it to reflect the powers that the goddess Mother Nature confers to us, it is necessary to prepare it for the exertion of practical magic.

Esoteric Works for Our Neighbor

Esoteric works for our neighbor are performed with the genii from the stars, with the elementals from Nature and with the "magic I." The magician's "magic I" is his Innermost.

For example: if we want to join an enamored couple in wedlock, we must beg our Innermost in order that He, in his turn, will beg Uriel. If Uriel allows this petition, then we will work with Uriel and with the elementals from Nature. Yet, if the petition to this genie from Venus is not accepted, then we have no other choice but to prostrate ourselves before the verdict of the law, because the law must not be violated. (Read the chapter entitled, "Astrotheurgy and Medicine").

While in meditation we can visit the Heart Temples of the stars, because through meditation we can achieve being completely within the Innermost. In other words, we can completely become the "superior I," who is the magic "I."

We can also visit the sidereal temples in our Astral Bodies.

The white magician does not violate the law. Whosoever performs magical works without permission of his Innermost and against the will of the divine hierarchies is a black magician who will pay his karma within the abyss.

Evil Eye on Children

I know of an unusual clinic in the town of San Luis de Cucuta.

In a very ancient, large, colonial style house, an old lady lives who knows how to cure the "evil eye." This house is always filled with mothers who carry their children in their arms so that this old lady can cure them from that sickness.

A certain person's child became sick and naturally this person took the child to the official physicians in order for them to prescribe a remedy for the child.

The physician's opinion was that the child was suffering from a stomach infection. Therefore, they prescribed him to fast and to drink boiled water as the only nourishment. Also, they prescribed him some powdered medicine within slips of paper and some liquid medicine, etc.

The result from all of this was worse. The child acquired great rings under his eyes. As well, fever, vomiting, and diarrhea were afflicting him.

Someone advised the child's father to take his sick son to that old woman's unusual clinic. So, when the old woman saw the child, she exclaimed, "An evil eye was placed on this child, which was caused by the sight of Mr. XX." Then, she added, "This child needs to be whispered to."

She took the little child in her arms and entered into her private room. The child was crying and screaming horribly.

The child's father became very worried while listening to the weeping of his son. Yet, some people advised him by saying, "You must not be afraid because the evil eye will leave the child through his weeping. You will see..."

Meanwhile, the old lady with the child in her arms appeared again in the room. The child was already healed.

The old lady spoke and said, "Your son is already healthy; two more whisperings and not even the roots of the evil eye will remain within him. Now you must bathe him in solar charged water within which you must place a piece of gold jewelry and a carnation."

The result was astonishing because the child became totally healed.

This old lady performed what all of those scoundrel-like impostors from the official medicine cannot do.

Another interesting case is the following:

A certain child of a physician from Cucuta became sick. That physician prescribed medicine by spoons, slips of papers, etc., to his own son. Yet, in spite of all this pharmacopoeia the sickness became worse. The worried physician resolved to call a reunion of physicians in order to search for a solution to this problem. However, all the remedies and all the theories of these physicians and his colleagues failed.

Then, the physician's wife, a little bit more "intuitive," resolved to take her child to this old woman. The result was astonishing. When seeing the child, the old lady said, "The child has received an evil eye."

Thus, the old lady whispered to the child and she healed him. The physician's wife told her husband what had happened and the physician himself paid the old lady for the healing.

What is curious in this case is that the mentioned physician kept in silence all that had happened. He never publicly spoke or wrote about it. This is because the false apostles of medicine feel shame when talking about these things. They are afraid to fall into ridicule. They are afraid of being qualified as "sorcerers" by the crowd.

This is how thousands of sick people die in the hands of these "foolish scientists" on a daily basis.

Formula in Order to Cure the Evil Eye

Obtain leaves of "oficion," leaves of "guandul" (*cajanus indicus [l.] Spreng*), "matarraton" (*gliricidia sepium [jacq.] Steud*).

These branches must be cooked in water and the child must be bathed in this decoction. The sick child is cured with three daily baths.

I know the case of a certain gentleman who has a terrible hypnotic power. It is enough for him to stare at a child and this child dies 24 hours later. That gentleman is conscious of his power. Therefore, he always avoids staring at children.

This occurs because the Ethereal Body of the child is more defenseless. Hence, it can be easily hurt by the hypnotic power of the people who have that power very well developed.

Reading from the four gospels depurates and cleanses the aura of people. Therefore, there are many curanderos who cure these cases by reciting from the four gospels and blessing the child with the sign of the cross.

Coral, gold, and jet (hard, black variety of lignite) assist the children against the evil eye.

Cases of Psychic Possession

The Bible describes innumerable cases of possessed people. Sage and rue plants were utilized abundantly in the Middle Ages in order to combat the evil entities that possessed people. The smoke from these plants was utilized.

Sage is one of the most efficient plants in order to combat cases in which the body of a person is possessed by an evil entity that obsesses the person and even makes him demented.

The elemental of the sage uses a pale, yellow colored

tunic, and has the marvelous power of healing the possessed.

This plant must be harvested during the night. First, it must be blessed, then it must be yanked by surprise from its very roots. The plant must be crushed, and the pressed juice is given to the possessed one to drink. Its leaves can also be pressed within water, and this water is then given to the possessed one to drink.

The plant must be burned so that the smoke may be utilized for the possessed one. The smoke from the plant must cover him. The evil entity must be conjured with an exorcism.

A gadget made with long pieces of glass and the exorcism from a secret book was employed in ancient times. However, the Conjuration of the Four can be used today.

Conjuration of the Four

> *Caput mortum, imperet tibi dominus per vivum et devotum serpentem!*
>
> *Cherub, imperet tibi Dominus per Adam Yod Havah!*
>
> *Aquila errans, imperet tibi Dominus per alas tauri!*
>
> *Serpens, imperet tibi Dominus Tetragrammaton, per Angelum et Leonem!*
>
> *Michael, Gabriel, Raphael, Anael!*
>
> *Fluat udor per Spiritum Elohim!*
>
> *Manet in terra per Adam Yod-Chavah!*
>
> *Fiat firmamentum per Yod Havah-Sabaoth!*
>
> *Fiat judicium per ignem in virtute Michael!*
>
> *Angel of the blind eyes, obey, or pass away with this holy water!*

SAGE

Work winged bull, or revert to the earth, unless thou wilt that I should pierce thee with this sword!

Chained eagle, obey my sign, or fly before this breathing!

Writhing serpent, crawl at my feet, or be tortured by the sacred fire, and give way before the perfumes that I burn in it!

Water, return to water!

Fire, burn!

Air, circulate!

Earth, revert to earth!

By virtue of the Pentagram, which is the morning star, and by the name of the Tetragram, which is written in the center of the cross of Light!

Amen. Amen. Amen.

It is necessary to seat the possessed one on a chair and to draw a circle around him on the floor with a piece of charcoal. Also, the Tetragrammaton [יהוה]—a sign in front of which all the columns of demons flee terrorized—must be drawn on the floor with charcoal at the threshold of the room (inside the room at its entrance).

The two vertexes (feet) of the star of five points or Pentagram will be aiming towards the outside of the room and the superior vortex (head) will be aiming towards the inside of the room. See the figure of the Pentagram:

The magician must magnetize the patient with the firm resolution of casting the possessing entity out from him. Yet, he must never hypnotize the possessed one, because hypnosis is purely and undeniably black magic.

The magician must conjure the possessing entity with the empire of his whole might. He must hold in his hand a sword or a knife with a new handle in order to imperiously command the perverse entity. This is done with the goal of terrorizing it, so that it will abandon the body of its victim.

The elemental of the sage plant must be commanded to eject the evil entity out of the body of the victim and to keep him in custody for an unlimited time.

When the victim is freed from the perverse entity that was obsessing him, then it is necessary to capture the perverse entity in order to prevent it from returning again inside his victim. Therefore, the medic magician must perform the ritual of the "bejuco de cadena" (*Bauhinia excisa Hemsl.*). This ritual must be practiced in the following way:

Bless the "bejuco de cadena" and command its elemental to enclose the perverse entity. Then, cut two lianas (bejucos) and put them on the floor forming a cross, and trace a circle on the floor around the cross in order to form our famous Gnostic circle, which is the cross within the circle of eternity.

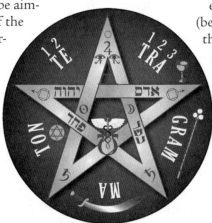

THE PENTAGRAM

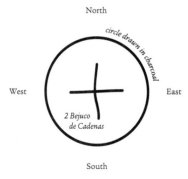

Then, the magician walks on the floor over the traced circle. He must start walking from south to north around the circle in order to return to the south again. One must follow the course of the circle by walking on its right side.

The two "bejucos de cadenas" that form the cross will mark the south and the north, the east and the west. Therefore, they will be placed in accordance with the four cardinal points of the earth.

When the magician finishes his revolution around the circle, as we already stated always walking towards its right side, then the magician will pass through the center of the circle from south to north, after having cut the center of the horizontal liana (bejuco) into two branches.

After having reached the north of the circle, the magician will walk towards the east of the circle, always walking on the right side of it. Once he is there, he will cut the other liana (bejuco) in the same way as he did the first one, and will resolutely pass through the center of the circle from east to west, thus moving forward without looking anywhere else. The perverse entity will remain enclosed in the center of the circle and in this way that entity will not return inside of his former victim.

The elemental from the "bejuco de cadena" uses a yellow tunic and is very intel-

ligent. He observes the ritual in silence. Then, he revolves around the circle while pronouncing his magical enchantments in order to apprehend the perverse entity.

The following graphic presents to us the steps of the magician when passing through the circle:

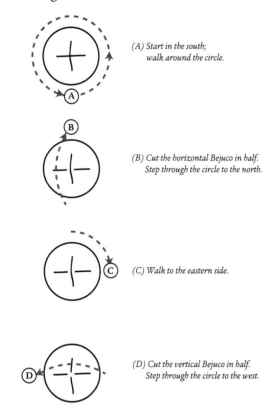

(A) Start in the south; walk around the circle.

(B) Cut the horizontal Bejuco in half. Step through the circle to the north.

(C) Walk to the eastern side.

(D) Cut the vertical Bejuco in half. Step through the circle to the west.

In this day and age, the "possessed people" go into hospitals for dementia, because the foolish scientists from this epoch are great charlatans who ignore these things.

With this clue, many possessed people can save themselves from going into hospitals for dementia. They die in those hospitals without those psychiatric doctors (who are praised because of their very boasted about "advanced methods") ever having the insight of investigating the cause of their illness.

There are many "crackbrain" spiritualists, morbid Theosophists, and sickening Rosicrucians everywhere who live comfortably in the great cities and who criticize the author of the present book and his profound studies regarding elementotherapy. Yet, none of them have had the patience of interning himself in the jungle in order to investigate the vegetal elementals.

How comfortable and how delectable it is to criticize while pleasantly seated and with quietude, without getting sunned or staying up all night in the jungle, without having to tolerate ants or venom, or poisons from ophidians!

Those so-called super-transcended ones are nothing more than "parasites" who live devouring the wisdom that the magicians acquired with supreme sacrifices. Thus, they devour it; not to comprehend, but to betray. This world is filled with social parasites and dim-witted critics.

Those super-transcended, foolish spiritists and spiritualists think that it is wrong to study the vegetal elementals without wanting to realize that the vegetal elementals are innocent angels and that in the epoch of Venus (the future cosmic day), they will be human beings and then later virtuous angels, solar pitris, and divine dyans.

We, the Gnostics, know very well that the elementals from the plants will be the human beings of the future.

Sicknesses Due to Consequences of the Will of Perverse People

If it is required to investigate the cause of a sickness that is suspected to be the conse-quence of witchcraft performed by the will of a perverse one, then a doll with bones of a rabbit, deer, black cattle, or tiger has to be carved. The bones must previously have been buried for a certain time. Thus, one must unbury them and make a doll as perfect as possible.

Build an altar with an arch in its farthest end. Utilize a branch of wild "totumo" (calabash tree, *Crescentia Cujete L.*) for the building of the arch. A branch from a sweet guava tree will serve for the cross of the altar. Place two flower vases and in each one of them a branch of the plant called bougainvillea or paper flower (*Bougainvillea glabra L.*).

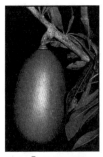 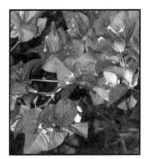

FRUIT OF THE CALABASH TREE.   BOUGAINVILLEA

The sick person must personally harvest the specified branches in the following ritualistic way: the branches from the "totumo" and guava by the eastern side and the bougainvillea by the western side.

The flower vases must be two crystal vases filled with water. A single branch of bougainvillea cut in two pieces will serve for each one of the two flower pots.

The altar must be built under a "guasimo" tree (*Guazuma ulmifolia Lamarck*). Pronounce the mantras of the "guasimo" tree and beg the elemental to show the sickness of the patient in the water of the flower vases. The mantras of the "guasimo" tree are:

Moud Mud Hammaca

The magician will remain kneeled before the altar. Then, after having made his petitions to the elemental of the "guasimo" tree, he will beseech the Angel Atan to intervene in order for the elemental to move the water and speak through the doll.

Have your sight fixed on the flower vases and observe what will appear in the water. If the sickness is due to magic from perverse wills, then the evil entities (the cause of the sickness) will be seen within the water.

Beseech the Angel Atan's assistance again and try to listen to the voice that comes out from the little bone figure; that voice will be clear and precise. Talk with it as if you were addressing a person.

The healing of the sick person will be made by the elemental of the "guasimo" tree. Pronounce the following healing mantras, while kneeling before the sick person:

Ae Gae Guf Pan Clara

Bless the back of the patient, perform magnetic passes, and give him the "guasimo" medicine to drink, which is the maceration of its leaves in rum for twenty days. DOSAGE: a little cup each hour.

The Master Huiracocha tells us extensively about these things in his *Initiatic Novel of Occultism* and in his book entitled *Sacred Plants*. Therefore, we do not say anything new, unreal, or fictitious. We only give details; we discover what is ignored.

Ceferino Maravita

One of the most astonishing medic-magicians from the Sierra Nevada of Santa Marta was the Indian Ceferino Maravita. Sick people who suffer sicknesses due to witchcraft must call every night to the "Mama" Ceferino Maravita, so he can cure them from their illness.

The following invocation must be performed:

> *In the name of Kalusuanga, the primeval god of light, son of the seven red seas and of the seven rays from the Sun, I invoke Thee, Mama Ceferino Maravita, so Thou can cure me from my illness. Amen.*

Curative Words (Mantras)

I disagree with the magician Omar Cherenzi Lind when he affirms in his book entitled *AUM* that the whole power of the verb is found in the silence, and that the verb must be silent. That gentleman wants to deprive us of the sublime and grandiose power of the articulated word. He ignores that the verb is of triple pronunciation and that it endows three norms: verbal, mental, and conscious.

One can articulate with the creative larynx, one can vocalize with his thought, and one can vocalize with the superlative consciousness of the Being.

We speak about the great creative verb, and we teach humanity the secrets of the creative word in our book in preparation entitled *Logos Mantra Theurgy*.

There are words that cure and words that kill. The physician's words are life or death for the sick person. A great amount of the physician's responsibility lies in their words, whether they employ their verb for constructive or destructive goals. No sick person should ever feel hopeless or condemned.

The physician must always say to his sick patient, "You are improving," "You are being healed," "Your healing is increasing," "Your sickness is disappearing," "Soon you will be better," etc.

These phrases are recorded within the subconsciousness of the sick person. Consequently, the sick person will be rapidly healed. No matter how grave a patient might be or looks to be, the condition of his health must never be revealed as delicate or dangerous, etc. With these negative and destructive words, death is accelerated for the patient. When the patient is addressed with contrary terms, with words of hope and strength, his health can totally improve and be cured.

There are words to cure the sick person, and magnetism combined with the verb becomes astonishing.

The morbid fluids of the sickness must be taken away with great flowing passes; that is to say, the morbid fluids of the sickness must be taken away from the head towards the feet. While they are being extracted, they must be burned within the fire of a lit candle or within charcoal embers.

Afterwards, Prana or magnetic vitality must be administrated over the solar plexus and over the sick organs with slow magnetic passes and with magnetic insufflations.

The magnetic insufflations are performed by inhaling oxygen and Prana and, after having mentally charged it with our vitality, it must be exhaled within a handkerchief and applied over the sick organs of the patient. This act must be accompanied with a powerful concentration of the will and the imagination, united in a vibrating harmony.

The physician will imagine the patient swimming within a blue-colored sea, and will pronounce the following mantras or magical words:

Ae Gae Guf Pan Clara
Aum Tat Sat Pan Tan Paz...

Ae Gae are gutturally pronounced by uniting the A with the E in a single sound, vocalized with the throat. (The "A" is pronounced as in the word "at" and the "E" as in the word "end").

The monosyllable **AUM** is pronounced *aom*. Open your mouth very well with the A, round your mouth with the O, and close your mouth with the M, like this:

Aaaaaaaaaaaaaaaaa
Ooooooooooooooo Mmmmmmmm

All of these mantras possess great healing powers. The masters from the White Fraternity must be invoked in order to cure the sick people.

The venerable master from the White Fraternity (Huiracocha) wrote in some Gnostic rituals certain mantras in order to invoke the masters. Let us see some of them.

E.U.O.E.	*I.A.O.*
Ischurion	*Athanaton*
Abroton	*E.U.O.E.*
I.A.O.	*Sabaoth*

Others are as follows:

Kirie Mitras	*Kirie Phalle*
Hagios	*Hagios*, **etc.**

The mantra **Hagios**, among other things, has the power of opening the whole atmosphere in order for the master to come.

Really, these mantras are good for that purpose. However, there are other more simple, efficient and at the same time shorter mantras in order to invoke the masters. Those mantras are the following:

Antia Da Una Sastaza

These mantras must be sung when pronounced. After having articulated them, the name of the master one wants to invoke has to be pronounced three times. Sick people can invoke the Master Hippocrates, father of medicine, or Galenus, Paracelsus, Hermes Trismegistus, etc.

The vowels **I.E.O.U.A.** have great healing powers:

1. The vowel **I** makes the blood rise towards the head. It cures the organs of the brain and develops clairvoyance.

2. The vowel **E** makes the blood rise towards the larynx. It cures sicknesses in the larynx and develops the magic ear.

3. The vowel **O** carries the blood to the heart. It cures this organ and awakens in us the sense of intuition.

4. The vowel **U** carries the blood to the solar plexus (tip of the stomach). It awakens the sense of telepathy and heals the stomach.

5. The vowel **A** carries the blood to the lungs and grants us the power of remembering our past reincarnations. At the same time, it heals the lungs.

These vowels are vocalized in combination with the letter **N**, like this:

IiiiiiiiiiiiiiiiiiiiiiiiiiiiNnnnnnnnnnnn

EeeeeeeeeeeeeNnnnnnnnnnnn

OooooooooooNnnnnnnnnnnn

UuuuuuuuuuuNnnnnnnnnnnn

AaaaaaaaaaaaNnnnnnnnnnnn

One hour daily of vocalization throughout our life makes us magicians. One can vocalize with the larynx, with the mind, with the heart, by meditating in the forces of these five vowels, such as we taught in the former pages.

There are certain mantras in order to awaken the chakras or esoteric powers. These mantras are based on these five vowels. These mantras are the following:

1. **SUIRA** (middlebrow) clairvoyance
2. **SUERA** (larynx) magic ear
3. **SUORA** (heart) intuition
4. **SUURA** (solar plexus) telepathy
5. **SUARA** (lungs) power to remember past incarnations

The correct pronunciation of these powerful mantras is in the following way:

Suuiiiiiiiiiiiiiiii Raaaaaaaaaaaaa

Suueeeeeeeeeee Raaaaaaaaaaaaaa

Suuooooooooo Raaaaaaaaaaaaaa

Suuuuuuuuuu Raaaaaaaaaaaaaa

Suuaaaaaaaaaa Raaaaaaaaaaaaaa

By means of these mantras, we carry the fire from our solar plexus towards all of our chakras in order to animate and awaken them. It is good to emphasize the importance of prolonging the sound of these vowels.

Sicknesses of the Mental Body

The Mental Body is a material organism that has its anatomy and its esoteric ultraphysiology.

The mantra in order to cure the sicknesses of the Mental Body is:

S M Hon

The **S** is pronounced as a piercing hissing sound, similar to the sound produced by brakes of compressed air, like this: *Ssssss sssssssssssssssssssssssss...*

The **M** is pronounced as when one imitates the bellow of the oxen: *Mmmmmmmmmm...*

The **H** is like a deep sigh. The syllable **ON** is pronounced by elongating the sound of the **O** and the **N**, like this: *Oooooo oooooooooooNnnnnnnnnnnnnnnnnn...*

This mantra must be vocalized daily for one hour. The disciple must invoke daily the Archangel Raphael and Hermes Trismegistus, supplicating them to heal his Mental Body.

When the sicknesses of the Mental Body crystallize in the physical brain, then madness is the outcome.

We study within the supra-sensible worlds the anatomy and physiology of the internal bodies of the human being.

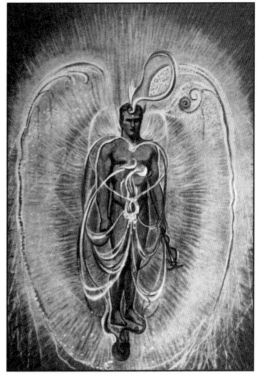

THE SILVER SHIELD OF THE MENTAL BODY AS ILLUSTRATED IN "THE DAYSPRING OF YOUTH" BY M.

Secrets of Practical Magic

Folklore from the Sierra Nevada

Many wise Indians are venerated in the Sierra Nevada of Santa Marta (Colombia). In cases of grave sicknesses, we can call them with our thought and our heart. Let us see a list of these wise Indians:

"God Kogi" (Mamankú)

"Mama" Yuisa Quintana Ríual

"Mama" Iskaviga

"Mama" Rayintana

"Mama" Marrocorrúa

"Mama" Cajaka

The "Saga" Catalina Alberto

The "Saga" Sinkiri

The "Saga" Yuila

"Mama Serancua"

These wise Indian medics live in the Astral Plane, and they come to the bed of the sick person who calls them with his thoughts and heart filled with faith.

There is a small temple in Buringueca where the Indians "pay" the Goddess Mother of the world (Nature) by carrying offerings to her.

There is a temple in Jinn State where the degree of "Poporo" is attained. This temple is called "Sokarua" (from Yoburo).

There are also temples in Jinn State in Garua and Gamaque. The temple of "Guicanuma" is also very important.

Therefore, the Sierra Nevada from Santa Marta is the "Tibet" of Colombia. The Indians adore Blessed Nature. They worship and bring offerings to her.

In the temple of Tierra Nueva, they often use in their worship a very important relic, which is called "gurrumaya." It is a relic of Cansamaria or Concoruba, which is a seashell in the form of a small plate or small cooking pan.

There are many marine shells that the Arhuacos use in their worship. Romantically, they call the Caribbean Sea "macuriba." The seashells that they use in their temples are called "chengues," which they have qualified into four types: red chengue, yellow chengue, black chengue, and white chengue.

These four colors remind us of the four races that have existed in the world:

1. Red race (Native American red skinned people)

2. Yellow race (Asiatic people)

3. Black race (African people)

4. White race (Occidental people)

These four races are symbolized by the four horses from the sacred scriptures (Revelation).

There is a small fruit called "gulaba" that the Arhuaco Indians employ in their worship to pay the blessed Goddess Mother of the world, Goddess Nature (Isis, Adonia, Insoberta, Mary).

There is another small fruit called "seitamaca," which also has great esoteric powers and is very sacred for them. The "concalva" is a big fruit from the Sierra Nevada, which they use in their sacred rituals.

The sacred rituals of the wise Arhuaco Indians and their wise utilization of the elementals allows them to control the Tattvas, although only in a partial form. This is because the mastery over the

Tattvas can only be achieved by the adepts of the White Fraternity. However, there are also adepts from the White Fraternity among the initiates of the Mayan Ray.

The founder of the College of Initiates is the "Maha-Guru" who dwells in Eastern Tibet. We, the masters of the White Lodge, achieved the mastery over the Tattvas. We converted ourselves into kings and queens of creation after we fused ourselves with our

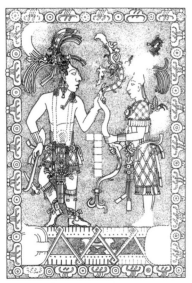

THE MAYAN SNAKE DANCE

Innermost (Spirit), also after we redeemed our animal soul. This is accomplished by assimilating the psychic extract of the Ethereal Body, the psychic extract of the Astral Body and the psychic extract of the Mental Body, within our Spiritual Soul.

We have two souls, which are mentioned by Goethe in his *Faust*. These are the animal soul and the diamond soul. The beautiful Sulamite (diamond soul) is betrothed with Solomon (the Innermost) when one achieves high initiation. This is how the Soul and the Spirit are fused and become "one."

Afterwards, the adept has to liberate his animal soul by assimilating the psychic extracts from his Ethereal, Emotional (Astral), and Mental bodies, so that he can verify the Ascension of the Lord, which is the fusion with the Glorian. This is how the master is transformed into a divine angel, into a medic of the Light, and into a theurgist.

The Divine Rabbi from Galilee practiced the Gospel and healed the sick because he was a true magician and theurgist, a true god.

"Magic" comes from *mag*, which means "priest." It signifies great power from the divine wisdom, the ineffable Light, the solar substance that the medic magician manipulates in order to heal those who are ill.

When the human being fuses himself with his own Innermost, he converts himself into a god of Nature. This is why the masters from the Mayan Ray are ineffable gods of Nature.

Introduce the virile member into the feminine vagina and withdraw it without spilling the semen (without reaching the orgasm). Whosoever renounces fornication and practices this secret daily, living a holy life, will also be converted into a god of Nature and into a medic-magician.

We also will become gods by becoming initiates of the "green snake." The priests of the snake were also venerated in Egypt.

Let us now see some gods or masters from the Mayan Ray, who are venerated by the Indians of the Sierra Nevada of Santa Marta (the "Tibet" of Colombia):

> Kakamulkuabi, a major secretary of the "Udumasi" hills, father of hailstorms.
>
> Sabatamena Laguna
>
> "Gualinutukua" is a temple where the Moors dance.
>
> Seyirico, "papa" of the "Jayo" (Mayan master)

The Master Ucua, mother of bon-cuá (the water).

The Master Abusudimba, mother.

There is a sacred temple called "Kembiterna" where the Moors dance. Another interesting temple is the one from Geingeka.

There is a sacred lagoon called "Sidigua." Pilgrims who walk towards the Indian masters who dwell in "Takima" and "Makutama" bathe themselves in this lagoon.

A very ancient dance called the "Cansamaria" is still danced in this day and age. The whole wisdom of these Indians is kept in secret behind the jagged mountain chain of the Paramos.

There is a sacred well and a guardian who remains seated in a certain place of the Sierra Nevada where the Mayan mysteries are cultivated. Those who are not prepared—that is to say, the unworthy—become enchanted when they arrive there... They cannot pass beyond this place.

The pilgrims bathe themselves in the lagoon in order to purify and cleanse themselves.

There is a temple called "La Gloria" at the shores of the Caribbean sea between Gaira and "Pozos Colorados."

The masters from the Mayan Ray are true dragons of wisdom, initiates of the snake. All of the inventions from Atlantis and Lemuria are kept as sacred relics in the temple of Kalusuanga, the Son of the Seven Red Seas and of the Seven Rays of the Sun. He is a Mayan master.

The Arhuaco Indians know in depth about the esoteric powers of the marine snail-shells. They use them as amulets.

COCA USE IN AN INCAN ARTIFACT (DATE UNKNOWN).

The "muchulo" is a marine shell with the shape of the feminine genitalia. There are large and small sizes that are carried around the necks by the female Indians. The large shells are for the women and the small shells for the girls. The esoteric powers of these snail-shells assist these female Indians against the sly and perverse fornicators.

There are certain snail-shells with the shape of cartridges, which are called "deriches" by the Indians. There are large and small sizes. The small ones are carried around the necks of the boys and the large ones are used by the men. These snail-shells assist them against witchcraft and evil entities.

The Arhuaco Indians always carry two "calabacitos" (calabash) when they travel through their mountains. They also chew coca leaves ("jayo") and dab a small stick within a "calabacito" with "ambira." Then, they put the stick into the other "calabacito" with marine shell flour. They carry this small stick in order to dab the coca ("jayo") with these, so they may perform long walks without getting tired, because the marine shells totally re-calcify them. Thus, when the osseous system is re-calcified in this way, it tolerates long walks.

There are also perverse black "Mamas" in the Sierra Nevada of Santa Marta who are capable of all type of evilness, since there are many things existing in the world.

In eastern Tibet, there are many Mahatmas. However, many Drukpas* and Böns* of the Red Hat also live there who

* Upon further investigation, the author corrected this statement by saying that the Böns are not necessarily black, just extreme in their efforts. Also see "Drukpa" in the Glossary on page 224.

are capable of all mischief and evilness, since they are black magicians.

There is a gigantic and very ancient city called "Maoa" in the flatlands of Casanare (Colombia). That city is in the Jinn state. This city will never be found by the "civilized" ones.

There is also another city in Jinn state in the Florida peninsula. This city will also never be found by the civilized ones.

There are secret cities in California that are inhabited by Lemurians, who are survivors from the continent "**Mu**."

There is a subterranean city under the thick jungles of the Amazon. Enormous riches from the Atlanteans are held here. This city is also inhabited.

The medical wisdom is preserved in all of these cities and Jinn lands. Lawfully, their inhabitants have the right of laughing about the "university horses" from our faculties of medicine.

The Egyptians mummified their cadavers. This mummification was performed by introducing the deceased person's Ethereal Body within his physical body. This is how the Ethereal Body suspended the decomposition of the cadaver.

When the "**Nous**" atom leaves the left ventricle of the heart, then the atoms of death direct the process of disintegration of the cadaver, and the physical body disintegrates. Thus, each atom has its own intelligence. These atomic angels have also soul and body, because each atom is the body of an atomic angel.

The Egyptians were suspending the work of the atoms of death by introducing the "Nous" atom within its sanctuary again. This sanctuary is situated in the left ventricle of the heart.

Nevertheless, the mummies from the Arhuaco Indians are much more perfect, because in addition to the mummification of the cadaver, they were "reducing" those cadavers to the size of small Lilliputians, and conserving perfectly the features of those cadavers.

Still, in this day and age, the "foolish scientists" from the official medicine cannot mummify a cadaver because they do not know the internal anatomy of the human being. The embalming of a cadaver can never be coequal to a mummification work, because the mummy is very much perfect.

As well, the modern scientists have not invented a remedy in order to preserve the youth and the life of the physical body for an unlimited time.

Indeed, we, the Gnostic medics, have that secret. We know that the Count Saint Germain, who was mentioned by Giovanni Papini, lives in Tibet with the same body which he used in the seventeenth, eighteenth, and nineteenth centuries in Europe. This is because we, the Gnostic masters, can preserve the physical body for an unlimited time.

The Master Mejnour lived seven times seven centuries. Zanoni was initiated in ancient Chaldea and disincarnated by the guillotine during the French Revolution.

What do the foolish modern scientists know about this? The only thing that they want is money and more money.

The whole wisdom of the Arhuaco Indians is found behind the jagged mountain-chain of the Paramos. Yet, that wisdom will never be accessible to the civilized ones of this twentieth century.

The Indians who live in the lower part of the Sierra Nevada are ignorant. If the "foolish scientists" believe that those Indians know something, then they are very mistaken.

The true Mayan medical wisdom is only found behind the jagged mountain chain of the Paramos, and no profane one can enter into those temples of the Mayan Ray.

The masters from the Mayan Ray, the masters from eastern Tibet, the masters from the secret temple of Juratena in Boyacá (Colombia), have the authentic esoteric wisdom enclosed within their subterranean sanctuaries.

The distinct indigenous tribes of the whole world are the possessors of that archaic, ancient wisdom of the green snake.

The esotericism known in the cities is nothing but a grotesque caricature of the ancient wisdom hidden in the subterranean sanctuaries of the Andes, Bohemia, Tibet and in all the subterranean caverns of the Sierra Nevada of Santa Marta, in the Alps and the sandy deserts of Asia and Africa.

The authentic esoteric wisdom is found in Manoa, the secret city from the flatlands of Casanare, and in all the secret cities of the thick jungles of the whole world.

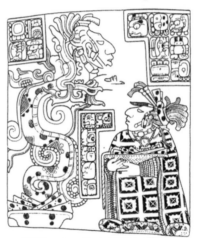

The Snake is the Giver of Wisdom. Mayan.

One needs to be humble in order to acquire wisdom, and after one has acquired it, there is the need to be even more humble.

I, Samael Aun Weor, the Avatar of the new Aquarian Era, am the first one teaching the ancient wisdom of the green snake to all the disciples who are lovers of the light.

The Gnostic Movement advances in a mighty way, and now nothing, not anyone, can stop us in this luminous and triumphal march.

The Snake and the Mirror

The "Saga" Maria Pastora is a great master from the Mayan Ray and a great illuminated sage in the powerful wisdom of the snake.

At present, the "Saga" lives on the greatest star of the "Great Bear." She never abandons her green snake.

The power of the medic-magician is based on the snake. The snake curanderos live making war amongst themselves. When a snake curandero has a lot of fame and clientele, then the rest of the curanderos make war upon him and they send serpents to bite him and kill him. Those snakes are sent abroad through the Astral Plane from far away. This is what we call Jinn state.

If the curandero is very well "sealed" with his Tattvic extracts, then he has nothing to be afraid of, because the viper's poison will not cause him any harm. Yet, if he is not "sealed," then inevitably he will die.

The snake curandero is a king within the vortex of the jungle, because nobody can cure the snake's bite but him. All the remedies from the pharmacy are worthless in these cases.

When a snake kills another snake, the victorious snake completely swallows the other. Afterwards, the snake vomits the other intact. Then, the victorious serpent searches for the leaves of a plant called "siempre viva" (*Sedum praealtum DC.*) and give these leaves to the victim to smell. Thus, the dead snake resurrects and runs away. The "siempre viva" plant is a liana that entangles itself everywhere and it has little leaves with the shape of a heart. It is the queen among all the plants that cure snake bites.

A circle must be traced around the plant before its harvesting. Then, it has to be blessed and one must beg the elemental of the plant for the services that one wishes from him, because it is not the plant that cures but its elemental.

Subsequently, the plant must be placed within a container with rum. Thus, when it is necessary to cure a person who has been bitten by a snake, this potion has to be given to him to drink and the area where the bite is found must be bathed with it.

The Indians are accustomed to always wear bracelets made with the skins of snake. The Arhuaco "Mamas" from the Sierra Nevada of Santa Marta remain entire hours sexually connected with their wives and they withdraw in the moment when they feel the approaching of the spasm, in order to avoid the spilling of the semen. In other words, they do not terminate the sexual act, because they suppress the orgasm. This is how they awake their "igneous snake."

On the rocky patios of the Aztec temples, young people from both sexes (couples) were naked, caressing each other, and connecting sexually. This was done during the period of entire months without ever consummating the sexual act (without reaching the orgasm). This is the way they transformed themselves into medic-magicians, by awakening the power of their igneous snake.

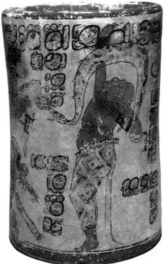

A JAGUAR-KNIGHT AND HIS SERPENT. MAYAN.

Within the mysteries of Eleusis, the sacred dance and Sexual Magic transformed human beings into gods.

The igneous snake is enclosed within a membranous bag that is situated in the coccygeal bone, which is the bone that serves as a base for the spinal column.

There is an ethereal chakra in the coccyx, and the spiritual fire snake resides there. When we practice sexual intercourse in the same way as the Arhuaco "Mamas" and the Aztec Indians, then this spiritual fire snake awakens and starts its ascension through the canal of the spinal column, until reaching the head.

When this spiritual fire snake reaches the head, then the Gnostic medic attains possession of all the powers of a god. He fuses himself with his Innermost, and becomes an angel. This igneous snake is called "Kundalini" by the Hindus.

The human being who has awakened his Kundalini becomes a physician anointed by God. The secret dwells in sexually connecting with our spouse and withdrawing from the sexual act without spilling the semen. Abundant information about this transcendental theme will be found in my books *The Perfect Matrimony* and *The Revolution of Beelzebub*.

Those who are awakening their igneous snake must help themselves with electric massages from the bottom to the top, along the spinal column. Any electric massage apparatus serves for this purpose.

While in the state of "Manteia" (ecstasy), the initiates can contemplate their resplendent Innermost, face to face, before the mirror of Eleusis. There is another marvelous mirror in the human being. The Gnostic medic must learn how to use this mirror by means of interior profound meditation... This mirror is imagination. For the wise ones, to imagine is to see. Imagination is clairvoyance itself.

Imagination is the mirror of the soul. It is the translucence through which we perceive the images from the Astral Light.

The Master Paracelsus states the following when he refers to the imagination:

> "The visible man has his laboratory (his physical body), and the invisible man works there. The Sun has its rays that are not possible to seize with the hands. Nevertheless, these rays are very strong (if they are brought together by means of a lens) and can burn edifices.

> "Imagination is like a sun, it operates within its own world wherever it glows. Man is what he thinks. If he thinks in fire, then he burns. If he thinks in war, then he is warring.

> "Imagination becomes a sun by means of the power of thought." - De Virtute Imaginativa

Imagination is developed by means of willpower. Willpower is invigorated and developed with imagination.

In order to magically operate upon the elementals of the plants and upon the organism of sick people, the Gnostic medic must unite his willpower and his imagination in a divine union.

Practice

The disciple must render himself daily to the practice of profound meditation. The theme of birth and death of plants is very simple as an exercise for interior meditation. The disciple must sit or lie down comfortably and stare for some moments at a plant, which he must already have for this exercise. He then closes his eyes and while preserving the image of the plant in his mind, he becomes somnolent. Once he is sleepy (somnolent), then he has to meditate on the growth of the plant from the time when it was a little, tiny stalk, until reaching its present state.

Remember that everything that is born has to eventually die. Imagine the plant in the process of decaying, withering, dying, converting into compost. Then, the disciple must fall asleep a little more and try to see and to converse with the elemental creature of that plant.

The elemental of that plant will be seen and heard after some time of daily practice. Then, the elemental will teach his secret formulae related with the sicknesses that he knows how to cure, and the elemental will place himself at the student's service for the execution of the works in which that elemental is an expert.

This medicinal procedure through interior profound meditation develops the disciple's own imagination. Thus, he will become an illuminated clairvoyant. He will direct his internal sight towards the most far away boundaries of the earth and will become a ruler of creation in its entirety. He will know the wisdom of each herb and thus he will unleash the tempests. He will transmute lead into gold and will make the earth tremble.

The fiery snake will make his mirror resplendent. Then, the disciple, abiding within his own cavern (his interior universe), will convert himself into a Dragon of Wisdom.

The magic of herbs allows us to unleash the waters and to make the entire universe tremble.

The Indians from the Sierra Nevada of Santa Marta preserve two cosmic books from very ancient times. One of them is called *El Anta*. Great cosmic powers are enclosed within these two books.

When we delivered to humanity our book entitled *The Perfect Matrimony*, which contains the most solemn message which the White Lodge has given to humanity since the first foundations of the world until our days were established, many passionate, perverted ones, mystical and sanctimonious people emerged who qualified us as pornographic. Those people took it personally. Thus, they cried... and vociferated in vain.

Some decrepit old men, who were rendered null because of too much copulation, declared that Sexual Magic was impossible. Thus, they pleaded for that absurd sexual abstention, for the unhealthy "chastity" of religious people. In other words, they pleaded for nocturnal pollutions, spermatorrhea, masturbation, and decalcification, because Nature cannot be violated with impunity. The sexual laws were not made in order to be transgressed.

To despise the woman—who is truly the best that man has, the most beautiful creature that life has granted—is a work of eunuchs, a work of masturbators, a work of sodomites. Woman converts man into an omnipotent god, who is capable of shaking the earth and unleashing lightning and tempests in the whole universe.

The "mystics" of Theosophy, the Rosicrucian Order, and Spiritualism called us "materialists." These offensive ones believed themselves to be super-transcendental, and they forgot that nothing can exist, not even God, without the help of matter. Sex is repulsive to them, but from where are they coming ? Who enrolled them in the school of life...?

Know then that initiation was not made for abnormal ones. Get ye hence, you eunuchs, sodomites, physically and morally decrepit ones...! Get ye hence, you fornicating spiritualists! Get ye hence, you classroom tyrants! The altar of initiation can only be approached by the true man and by the true woman.

My disciples must be intrepid, courageous, tenacious, ferrous, and of a character like a steel shield, always victorious, always rebellious as the heroic creations of the illustrious Rabelais.

Each one of my Gnostic disciples is a soldier in complete battle, in a field without boundaries, without parochial limitations, without compromises from sects and from lodges.

The Gnostic army is the army of Christ. The Gnostic army is now in battle against false religions, schools and sects from the world. It is against everything black, against everything that tastes of crime and exploitation.

The paladins from the new era emerge everywhere. We have Gnostic soldiers in the factories, in the workshops, in the ships, in the railroads, in commerce, in the banks, in industry, in the mines. In short, they are everywhere.

Now, not even one point more or one point less, whosoever is not with us is against us. We cannot tolerate more infamies and false promises from dim-witted politicians. Now we want to return into the fields of Nature in order to work. Now we want to return into the bosom of the blessed Goddess Mother of the world.

Now, we want a king, a president, a governor: Christ, Christ, only Christ!

Woe to those mystics who detest the woman! Woe to those passionate fornicators who only see in her an instrument of pleasure! Woeful ones... It would have been good for such men if they had not been born; or it would have been better for them if a millstone were hung about their necks, and they were drowned in the depth of the sea. [Matthew 18:6, Mark 9:42, Luke 17:2]

Whosoever wants to reach the altar of initiation has to thrust himself against his own defects, against his vices, in a battle face to face against the enemies who dwell in his own house (psyche).

Down with the chains of conventionalism! To the redeeming battle!

Secrets of the Magic Mirror

A mirror and three hairs from the crown of the head of an impressionable, nervous and sensitive woman must be placed in the bottom of a container with water. Then, the magician has to fixedly stare at the woman to whom he has to imperiously say: "Look, be well aware. Here, over this mirror is the image of (say here the name of the person who is going to be seen)."

Thus, the sensitive woman will do it, and she will see the desired person. If it is commanded, she will even see what the person is doing in that given moment.

The magician must magnetize the sensitive woman; yet, he must not hypnotize her, because hypnotism is black magic. The operator must invoke the Angel Anael, so that the angel can help him in this work. If

quicksilver is added to the water, then the result will be more effective.

The experiment will be performed within a dark room. A lit candle must be placed next to the container. It is convenient to smoke the room with frankincense and to conjure the evil entities with the Conjuration of the Four, as noted in the section entitled "Cases of Psychic Obsession." The sign of the Pentagram must be placed inside the room on the floor, at the door's entrance, as shown in the figure on page 53, in order to frighten away the infernal demons.

The woman for this type of work must be young, nervous, sensitive, and of a thin constitution. Heavy women are not suitable for this experiment. Thus, not all women are apt for certain psychic experiments.

Clairvoyance

Whosoever wants to become clairvoyant must reconquer the lost infancy.

The atoms of infancy live submerged within our internal universe and there is the necessity of putting them afloat again in order to attain divine clairvoyance. This labor can be performed by means of the verb. Therefore, the following mantras must be pronounced:

MaaaaaaaaaaaMaaaaaaaaaaa
PaaaaaaaaaaaPaaaaaaaaaaaa

These mantras must be sung by raising the tone of the voice with the first syllable of each word and descending the voice with the second syllable of each word. Then, the child who lives submerged within us emerges to existence again, and we become clairvoyant.

This teaching was delivered to me by the Angel Aroch, for the disciples. These exercises of vocalization must be practiced daily.

Teachings of Christ

Christ taught a great mantra in order to cure the deaf and those who stutter:

> **EPHPHATHA** ("Be opened"), see Chapter 7 verses 32-37, Gospel of Saint Mark.

Another very interesting mantra taught by Christ in order to cure the sick and to resurrect the dead is the following: **TALITHA CUMI**. Is this difficult? Resurrection is only possible when the silver cord has not been cut. In such cases, heat must be breathed into the lips of the cadaver. The defunct must be taken by the hand. Then, the mantra *Talitha Cumi* must be pronounced and the name of the deceased has to be called three times.

This very high magical work is only possible when the Law permits it.

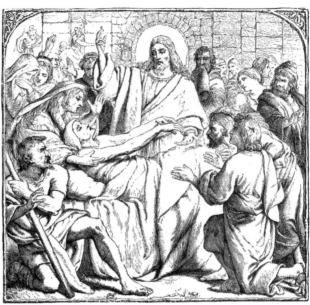

A Curious Case

On a certain occasion, a curious case occurred in Barranquilla (Colombia). A girl became gravely sick. Official science could not cure her. The girl presented the following symptoms: vomiting, diarrhea, and she was becoming thin in general, accompanied by extreme weakness.

Official physicians proceeded as is customary. They administered penicillin, serum, etc., without any results. Afterwards, while conversing in detail with the girl's mother, they became aware that the mother was breastfeeding her girl, in spite of being pregnant again.

The mother was pregnant with a baby of the masculine sex and logically, her breast milk was not suitable for a child of the opposite sex, because the constitution of the mother's milk is different in each case.

Therefore, a meeting of physicians took place and they arrived at the conclusion that the improper milk should be eliminated from the girl's sick organism. Thus, they proceeded as customary, with innumerable remedies and prescriptions that instead of curing the girl, were making her organism worse.

Then, somebody informed the physicians that an Indian was in the city who knew a great deal about medicine. So, the Indian was called by the physicians. He entered into the room of the sick girl while those doctors were still meeting around the bed of the sick girl. The Indian (a native from the state of Bolivar, Colombia) saw the girl and said: "This girl has been nourished with bad milk from a pregnant woman. However, I am going to take the milk from her body at once." Consequently, he sent a boy to his house to bring him a determined medicament.

The Indian gave the girl the remedy to drink and after a few minutes, the girl felt the necessity of evacuating. When performing this physiological function, the girl excreted the faulty milk before the sight of the astonished physicians, who, with pencils in their hands, were asking the Indian for the medicament's formula. Yet, after showing them the faulty milk within a bottle, the Indian looked at them with the most profound despise and left that home without the astonished physicians learning about the mysterious formula.

The girl was totally healed and medical science was totally mocked.

Later on, the Indian did not have any trouble in revealing the formula to me. This formula is as follows:

> Obtain colostrum from the breast of a woman whose child is of the same sex of the sick child. This must be mixed with the milk of the "Perrillo" tree which is a very well known tree in Antioquia (Colombia).

Indication:

If the child is male and he drank milk from a pregnant woman whose pregnancy is of a female fetus, then the colostrum of another woman who is nourishing a boy will be given to the sick male child, and vice versa: if the sick child is a girl, then colostrum from another woman who is nourishing a baby girl is used.

The Gnostic medic must always have these remedies previously prepared.

Disincarnation

When that which is called death occurs, then the ego abandons the physical body. The ego or soul is united to the physical body through the silver cord. This cord of astral matter is the one that maintains the soul united to the physical body. Yet, when that cord is cut, then the soul can no longer enter into the physical body. Commonly, that cord is cut three days after death has occurred.

The silver cord is united to the left ventricle of the heart. When we travel in the Astral Body, the soul can return into the physical body thanks to that cord. However, when death occurs, the soul can no longer return into her physical body, because the cord is already cut.

In the last moments of life, the dying person sees the angel of death as if he was a skull or a spectral being. The angel of death, or angels of death, are perfect beings whose mission is to take the souls out of their bodies in the supreme instant of death.

These angels of death have to cut the silver cord and their intervention is always sensed by those who are dying. Once this work is done, the angel withdraws and the soul of the deceased continues living in the same environment. However, we have to declare that an irresistible fluidic attraction continues to exist between the soul and the body after death.

Commonly, the souls of the dead that are attracted by their physical bodies, which are in the process of decomposition, inundate the graveyards or cemeteries. This is why cemeteries have a horrible appearance before the sight of the exercised clairvoyants.

The deceased ones mold the astral part of their tombs by means of their imagination. Thus, they give to their tombs the aspect of bedrooms or hospital rooms. The astral matter is essentially flexible. Therefore, that matter takes any form that the imagination gives it. For example, if you, beloved reader, imagine a hat, then that hat will be converted into a reality in the Astral World.

Accordingly, by means of the Astral Light and their imagination, the souls of the dead give their tombs the same appearance as their room, sleeping compartment, or the room in which they were in their last days. This is because the image of that bedroom is strongly recorded in their minds.

The cadaver attracts the soul and the soul acts upon the plastic matter of the Astral World by means of the imagination. This is how the soul transforms the tomb into a bedroom or into a hospital room.

The exercised clairvoyant can see the souls of the dead walking by in the cemeteries. They talk about their sicknesses, about their bitterness, about a possible healing, about medicines, etc.

Before the imagination of the souls of the dead, the cemetery is not a cemetery. For them the cemetery is hospitals, halls, bedrooms, clinics, etc. Each tomb is for them a hall, a clinic, a bedroom, etc. Those souls still believe they are in flesh and bones. Therefore, they feel the same sicknesses that were the cause of their death.

Commonly, those souls exhale the filthy smell of their cadaver in putrefaction. Those souls suffer the same bitterness of

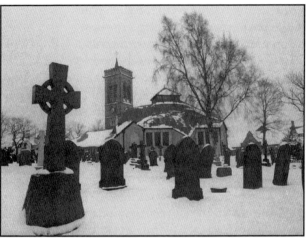

A GRAVEYARD IN THE UNITED KINGDOM.

their former life. Thus, they hope to be healed from their sicknesses.

This horrible attraction of the souls towards the cemeteries disappears as soon as the cadaver has become ashes. Hence, when the cadaver is already ashes the soul feels healed and happy and abandons the cemetery, which, with her turbid imagination, she believed to be a clinic, rooms, halls, hospitals, etc.

Nevertheless, if the cadaver is burned, then, the soul avoids passing through all those horrible sufferings in the cemetery.

Therefore, for charity, for compassion, for pity and for love towards our beloved, the cadavers must be burned, because suffering within cemeteries is horrible.

It is very hard for a soul to live within a tomb that is believed to be a hall or bedroom. This is the cause of the horror that the living ones have towards the cemeteries, because as long as the body continues existing, it will attract the soul towards the tomb, and the soul will suffer the unutterable.

It is a thousand times preferable to pass through the pain of burning the cadaver of a beloved defunct, than to leave his poor soul to be tormented within a cemetery.

You must be compassionate towards your beloved relative. Burn his cadaver, so that the soul can be liberated from the horrible bitterness of the cemetery. You must not be cruel with your beloved relative, so burn the body in order for that beloved soul to be free from the cemetery.

What has been explained about the cemeteries is what has been experienced by some seers.

When I was in the city of Pamplona (north of Santander, Colombia), I knew about an interesting case related with this theme about which we are commenting.

On one of those solitary and cold nights, a certain gentleman, whose name I do not want to mention, was walking through a street of that city that is surrounded by paramount hills.

Then, this gentleman saw a beautiful lady. With compliments, he offered to accompany her to her house. The lady inflamed upon this gentleman the desire of an intimate relation and she did not reject his company.

Thus, this fellow was happily walking with the lady while longing for a romantic Don Juan-type of adventure.

Suddenly, the lady stopped before the elegant door of a luxurious mansion that was surrounded by magnificent gardens. Then, sweet words and lovely phrases were uttered there. Finally, the lady invited the enamored gentleman to enter inside her enchanted dwelling. Feeling himself happy, this handsome man, who was filled with an irresistible sexual desire, entered into that beautiful lady's bedroom.

The enamored man lay down over the improvised nuptial bed and he fell asleep there without the lady lying herself next to him.

When this handsome man awoke, the Sun was already illuminating the vast horizons and the humid summits of those paramount hills that surround Pamplona city. He felt a little bit uncomfortable in the bed and he saw that the walls of that room were menacingly closing themselves over him. "Where am I?" he asked himself. "Where is that lady?"

Then, by meticulously staring around him, he saw with horror that he was inside a large tomb of the cemetery. He could not utter a word. He became filled with a horrible panic and collapsed. Several hours later, some visitors found this gentleman within that tomb and subsequently, they took him unconscious out of the tomb.

After medical intervention, the gentleman recuperated his lucidity and told the authorities all that had occurred. Naturally, the authorities declared that he was insane.

Many years ago, a cadaver of a beautiful lady had been buried within that tomb. Yet, the lady with her imagination within the Astral Plane had converted that tomb into an elegant mansion. Undoubtedly, she was already liberated from the attraction of that cadaver. However, she was not free from the attraction towards that beautiful mansion constructed by her in the Astral Plane or within the Astral environment of that tomb.

The lady took this gentleman out from this chemical region (physical dimension) and thus, she placed his physical body and the whole of him inside the Astral Plane. This is what is called in esotericism the "Jinn State."

Halls of Black Magic within Cemeteries

As strange as it may seem for many people, there truly exist halls of black magic within cemeteries, which are situated in the Astral Plane.

Those dismal halls respire all the rottenness from the burial grounds and the black magicians from those halls utilize all of those horrible elements from the cemetery for their infernal purposes.

Many astral vampires are within the astral environment of cemeteries. They nourish themselves from the cadaverous emanations and from the rottenness. Those vampires are utilized by the black magicians in order to cause harm to their hated enemies.

Since the earth inhales and exhales as we do, the soil from cemeteries constitutes great sources of infection for the urban populace. Great pestilence has gone out from cemeteries.

Typhus, variola, and all type of epidemic diseases have gone out from cemeteries.

The soil from cemeteries inhales oxygen and exhales epidemics. Scientists have already proven that the earth inhales and exhales. Therefore, our assertions are strictly scientific.

The hour has arrived in which the authorities of public health and sanitation must establish crematory furnaces instead of cemeteries.

The mourning relatives could establish in their homes altars where they can place the ashes of their beloved deceased relatives within beautiful and splendid "coffins." Thus, the bonds between the ascendants and descendants will be maintained through those ashes.

Within the halls of black magic in cemeteries, a true swarm of perverse entities and malignant atoms are available to the black magicians in order to perform their operations of black magic.

Those black magicians recruit millions of perverse souls whose bodies have been buried in cemeteries, in order to put them to work under their command. All such actions make the cemeteries not only sources of physical epidemics, but also sources of moral epidemics.

Each atom is a trio of matter, energy, and consciousness—that is to say, each atom is an atomic intelligence. Therefore, the atoms from criminals and evil ones who are buried in the cemeteries constitute true moral epidemics, which are specifically concentrated within the cemeteries.

The atoms that we inhale in the cemeteries enter our organism, and they form evil communities within the space that separates the objective system from our secondary system or grand sympathetic system. These atomic, evil communities falsify our minds, and they invisibly float within our astral atmosphere. Thus, these atomic evil communities remain there, infecting us as a moral epidemic or as intelligences that excite us to perform all type of evilness.

Commonly, these colonies of evil atoms from cemeteries are more easily received inside the bodies of people during rainy weather.

The cemeteries are true infernos of evilness, weeping, and rottenness. The Ethereal Bodies of the deceased float as skeletons or horrible phantoms over and around the tombs. They constitute a fountain of spectral terror for the souls who are attracted to their physical bodies, which are in the state of decomposition within the burial grounds.

The Ethereal Bodies are simultaneously disintegrated along with the cadavers and they adopt their horrible spectral form. The tenebrous ones from the halls of black magic utilize those spectral phantoms in order to horrify the souls of the dead.

Moreover, these black magicians also utilize these spectral phantoms in order to frighten the living ones. There are innumerable cases of spectral apparitions that have been witnessed throughout time, in spite of the abundant mockery from ignorant chroniclers and superficial people of the epoch.

The phrase from the ignoramuses that states, "No one can know what happens in heaven or of a supernatural nature," or, "No one knows what is in the other world, because no one has gone there yet," are truly phrases only among the fools from this epoch.

The Fourth Coordinate

Secret in Order to Function Within the Superior Vehicles

Every Gnostic medic must learn how to freely function in his Atmic and Buddhic vehicles in order to investigate the Nirvanic, Super-Nirvanic, Adic, Monadic, etc., planes.

The essences from superior planes are worthy of being studied. We can receive sublime teachings from the Buddhas of Contemplation while in Nirvana.

We can enter by will any time we want into those superlative planes of consciousness. The light of Atman the ineffable reigns there.

The disciple will start by learning how to depart from his physical body in his Astral vehicle.

Later on, when he is out of his body, he will beg his Innermost to take his inferior vehicles out from him. Then, his Innermost will take his Astral, Mental, Causal, etc., vehicles out from the atomic doors of his spinal column.

When we are without those inferior vehicles, we learn to move ourselves in the Buddhic and Atmic vehicles by will.

It is also true that in the Astral Body we can visit the Buddhic, Nirvanic, Adic, etc., worlds. The Theosophists do not know anything about this. Hence, they are worthy of pity.

It is also very true that through meditation we can visit the superior worlds. The Innermost can enter into any department of the kingdom.

The Mental World

Even though it seems incredible, black magicians also exist within the Mental World.

The black magicians from the Mental World are the most dangerous of the universe. Those black magicians from the Mental World are extremely fine, subtle, erudite, and delicate.

They can easily turn aside many investigators because they have the appearance of masters. When the master is christifying his Mental Body, then he has to confront great battles against these very dangerous adepts of the shadow.

The Mental Body is christified with the fourth degree of the power of the fire; that is to say, with the Kundalini of the Mental Body. Each one of our seven bodies has its own Kundalini.

The Mind

All the problems that we the human beings have to resolve, all the sufferings from our life, all our desires and passions, all our bitterness, reside within the mind.

If somebody throws a stone into a crystalline lake, then we will see a vast amount of waves that come from the center towards the periphery. These waves are the reaction of the water against the exterior impact.

Our mind is similar to this. The external impacts fall into the lake of our mind, which make us react towards the exterior world with waves of anger, desire, envy, slander, etc.

For example: When we see a pornographic illustration, this image strikes the retina of our eye. Afterwards, it passes towards our sensorial cerebral center, and finally it goes into our mind. Thus, our mind reacts over that exterior image with waves of carnal passion.

If somebody insults us, the insulter's words arrive to our senses, and afterwards they pass into our mind. Subsequently, our mind reacts with waves of fury and violence against the insulter.

Therefore, the mind is the cause of all our bitterness. It is the wild horse that hauls our wagon. If we do not dominate it with the whip of willpower, then it will haul our wagon into the abyss. The magician must manage his mind. The magician must dominate his mind by means of willpower.

When our mind is filled with passionate desires, then let us stop for a moment and let us imperiously command our mind as follows: "Mental Body, withdraw those thoughts from me. I do not allow you to bear them."

When our mind is filled with anger, then let us command our mind like this: "Mental Body, withdraw this anger from me. I do not allow you to bear anger."

When our mind is filled with hatred, then let us command our mind like this: "Mental Body, withdraw this hatred from me. I do not allow you to bear hatred, etc."

The Being is not the mind, the Being is the Being. He is the Innermost and He can control our mind by means of willpower.

The den of desire is within the mind. The body of desires is nothing but an emotional instrument of the mind.

We can converse with our mind in the internal worlds, when we momentarily have deprived ourselves from it.

Then, the mind seems to be almost an independent subject that sits in front of us, face to face, in order to converse.

This interesting experiment is performed in the following way:

1. The magician must abandon his physical body and depart within his Astral Body.

2. Once out, he must feel himself having a childlike heart.

3. Then, he must command his Astral Body as follows: "Astral Body, withdraw from me."

4. He must cast his Astral Body out from himself, through his spinal column.

5. Subsequently, his Astral Body will fall out of him from his back and will go out.

6. The disciple will remain within his Mental Body.

7. Now, he has to command his Mental Body as follows: "Mental Body, withdraw from me."

8. The disciple must throw his Mental Body out towards his back.

9. Now, the magician will feel that something else is moving within his own Being.

10. At this moment, a rare personage comes out from his spinal column.

11. The disciple must question this rare personage: "Who are you?"

12. This subject will answer as follows: "I am your Mental Body. Do you not know me?"

13. The disciple must now invite his own mind to sit.

14. This is now the precise moment in which the disciple can converse with his mind face to face, front to front.

After this profound investigation, the disciple will be aware that his mind is a wild horse, a savage man, which he must control, command, and direct with the whip of willpower.

All the torments of our existence come from the Mental Body.

No insults, no bitterness can ever reach our Innermost, because all bitterness, all insults only reach until the Mental Body. Therefore, it is only the mind that reacts towards the exterior world with tempests of pain and bitterness.

The Innermost cannot suffer. The Innermost suffers only when he identifies himself with his mind, when he still has not learned how to control his mind by means of his willpower.

The tempests of our existence come from the exterior, from the world of the mind. They do not come from within, from the profundities of the infinite, because there is where the Innermost always lives full of happiness.

Jinn Humans and Jinn Lands

Ms. Neel comments to us in a book about the semi-flying ascetics from Tibet who travel Tibet in all directions while in a type of somnambulistic dream state. They do this without eating or resting in any place. Their journeys last for many days, without them getting tired.

The peyote was utilized by the Aztec priests in their temples of mysteries in order to submerge the sick people into a profound dream, from which they were subsequently coming out from healed.

After a very profound dream, the mystos came out totally illuminated from the Greek, Toltec, and Egyptian temples.

Freud spoke to us about the tremendous energy of the subconsciousness and the Master Huiracocha taught us how to cure sick people with perfumes by taking advantage of a patient's dream.

This is because, in reality, the curative forces of the organism reside within the subconsciousness and the medic can manipulate them during the patient's dream.

The physician Dr. Schwab states that the brain and the nervous sympathetic plexus are the exponents of the curative force from the organism. He states that this plexus rules the involuntary functions and that it intervenes over the endocrine glands.

The subconsciousness is the base of the vital energies and the storage of all the forces.

A disciple of the "Mamas" named Juan Bautista Miranda lived in the state of Magdalena (Colombia). He cured cases of leprosy in the final stages and he made the scientists from the official medicine grow wan.

On a certain occasion, Miranda said to his people: "A sick person is near at hand in coming, but you must deny that I am here, otherwise I am lost." Subsequently, the sick person who was clairvoyantly predicted by this medic, arrived at the precise hour noted. Miranda's people tried to deny the medic's presence, yet the sick person answered: "The medic is here, and he must cure me."

This case was related to a work of witchcraft that Juan Bautista Miranda could easily cure. When the sick person was healed, then Juan Bautista Miranda became sick and he sent for his son. However, his luck was bad, because he died before his son's arrival.

The physical body of Juan Bautista Miranda was buried as is customary. Yet, the next day, the tomb was empty, as the cadaver had disappeared. What happened? Well, Juan Bautista Miranda lives in the Sierra Nevada from Santa Marta, performing marvelous healings. His death was only simulated, because the "Mamas" took his body from the tomb.

How did the "Mamas" take Juan Bautista Miranda's body? Dr. Steiner states that a physical body can remain within the internal worlds without losing its physical characteristics. This is what is called "Jinn State."

In the case of Juan Bautista Miranda, the "Mamas" operated by submerging his assumed dead body within the Astral Plane. This is how they transported him to the Sierra Nevada.

We know that there are fakirs in India who bury themselves alive and they endure months in this buried state. The case of Miranda was analogous.

When the Spanish Conquistadors came to America, the wise Indians hid their sacred temples by putting them into the Astral Plane. Those temples still exist in this day and age. However, they are hidden to the eyes of the profane. This is called "Jinn State."

Various of these esoteric (hidden) temples are in the Sierra Nevada from Santa Marta (Colombia). The "Mama" Matías, before his death, was officiating in "Pueblo Hundido" (sunken town) from the Sierra

Nevada. This "Mama" was asking forgiveness for his sick people and also health and life for them within that temple.

Another temple is the one in "Cheruba." The "Saga Catalina Alberto" officiated there.

The "Mama" Matías started to officiate in the temple of "Chinchicua" before his death.

All of these esoteric temples are called "temples from the god Nature" by the indigenous people.

Also in the Sierra Nevada there is a land in Jinn State where the black magistracy abides. It is called "Guanani." The river "Ariguani" runs there. The first door of this black magistracy is in a waterfall from this river. A huge dragon was seen there by the natives. The black magicians leave in the night through this door. All of these black magicians worship the demon "Ikanuse," who in this day and age has a physical body.

During a certain part of the year, the "Mamas" use special herbs in order to humiliate and defeat the black magistracy. They throw their bunches of herbs in that previously mentioned door. This is how they subdue these magicians from darkness.

There is an esoteric temple also in the mountain of Monserrate of Bogota, Colombia. Some Chibchas initiates dwell there. There are esoteric temples in the whole of South America.

Every student of Gnosticism has to learn how to transport himself in a few seconds towards his sick patients in order to visit and cure them. The procedure is in the following way:

The disciple must lie down on his left side with his head rested over the palm of the hand of the same side. Then, he has to get sleepy with his mind fixed in the process of the dream. Dream images emerge during the state of transition between vigil and dream. The disciple must reject such images, because if he does not do it, then he will remain abstracted within them and he will fall asleep.

The attention of the disciple must be fixed only and exclusively in the process of the dream. Then, when he feels that the dream has already invaded his brain, he must abandon all of his laziness and get up immediately. The whole secret of this matter rests in leaving our home, going out towards the street. Yet, we have to conserve the dreamy state.

When already on the street, the disciple has to jump with the intention of suspending himself in the air as if he was a bird. Then, he can transport himself in flesh and bones towards the residence of the sick person.

In this way, the disciple will learn how to travel in a few seconds to the most remote places of the earth in order to cure sick patients. He can also take his herbs and remedies with him.

The physical body enters, in this case, within the Astral Plane and remains out of the law of gravity. This process is performed by the powerful energies of the subconsciousness. This is why we insist that the disciple must leave his house while preserving his dreamy state.

The dream has its power and that power is the energies of the subconsciousness. It would be impossible for the physical body to enter into a Jinn State without the energies of the subconsciousness.

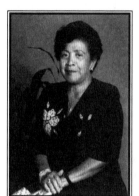

LITELANTES

The Master Litelantes, The Harpocranian Forces, the Orphic Egg, and the Jinn States

The Guru Litelantes, known on the Earth with the profane name of Arnolda de Gomez, taught me about the Jinn State.

This lady-adept is my priestess-wife and my esoteric collaborator.

I have read much esoteric literature, yet I have never found concrete data about the "modus operandi" for Jinn States.

The venerable Master Huiracocha relates to us in his *Initiatic Novel* the interesting case of the commander Montenero who, with his physical body in Jinn State, entered into the Temple of Chapultepec, Mexico, in order to receive cosmic initiation.

Don Mario Roso de Luna also speaks marvelously to us about the Jinn States.

However, never has any Spiritualist writer taught us the concrete formula in order to place the physical body in the Jinn State.

I learned this formula from my own priestess-wife. She taught it to me in a practical way. Regarding this, many interesting things from that time come into my memory.

Back in time, in the year 1946, my wife and I were living in the tropical town of Girardot (Cundinamarca). One certain day, the lady-adept told me, "Tonight I will transport myself with my physical body in Jinn State to the home of Mrs. E... I will make my appearance felt by her. Then, I will leave there a material object for her."

Being somewhat inquisitive, I asked her, "Is it possible to transport oneself with the physical body through the air and without the necessity of an airplane?"

While smiling, the Guru Litelantes told me, "You will see..."

The following day, very early, I went to visit Mrs. E... This lady, somehow overwhelmed, told me that during the whole night she had felt noise within her house and the steps of a strange person. Then, she told me that inside her home, which was properly closed with a lock, she had found certain material objects that belonged to Mrs. Arnolda.

I, overwhelmed from this matter, went to the lady-adept to tell her about the case. Smiling, she told me: "You see that it is possible to travel with the physical body in the Jinn State."

Later on, she invited me to execute an excursion with the physical body through the dominions of those marvelous Jinn lands that Don Mario Roso de Luna spoke about.

Hence, one night, the most quiet, the most silent night, I was lying down on my bed in a perfectly vigil state. Suddenly, the lady-adept told me: "Get up from your bed and let's go..."

This lady-adept had placed her physical body in Jinn State. Thus, she was surrounded by the tremendous cosmic forces from the God Harpocrates.

I got up from my bed and filled with faith I followed her, walking with a firm and decisive step. A spiritual volup-tuousness was inebriating me. So, I decided to float in the air. I comprehended that I had submerged myself within the Astral

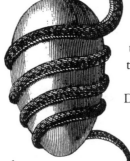

THE ORPHIC EGG

Plane, yet, I did it with my physical body. I understood that when the physical body is submerged within the Astral Body it can levitate and remain under the laws of the Astral Plane, yet without losing its physi-ological characteristics.

Once, while in Jinn State, the lady-adept made me fly over great precipices and mountains in order to prove my courage.

After having a very interesting excursion, which was performed in remote Jinn lands, the lady-adept and I returned to our dwell-ing.

I continued, experimenting on my own. Thus, I discovered that in order to trans-port oneself with the physical body in the Jinn State, only a minimum quantity of dream and a lot of faith is necessary.

Later on, the lady-adept explained to me something about the Orphic egg and the Jinn States.

The golden egg of Brahma, which symbolizes the universe, comes into my memory.

Our planet Earth has an oviform figure. The first manifestation of the cosmos in a form of an egg was the belief that was most spread in antiquity.

It is stated in the Egyptian rite that Seb, the god of time and the earth, laid an egg, or the universe; an egg that was brought into existence at the hour of the great ONE of the double force.

The God **Ra** is represented by the Egyptians in a process of ges-tation within an egg.

The Orphic egg appears in the Dionysian mysteries.

In Greece and India, the first visible masculine being who was reuniting the two sexes in himself was represented as emerging from an egg.

The egg symbolizes the world.

Therefore, logic invites us to think that great esoteric powers exist within the egg.

The Guru Litelantes explained to me the magic formula of the egg.

The Guru Litelantes told me that one can place the physical body in a Jinn State with the egg.

A small orifice must be made on the endmost pointed part of the egg. Then, the yolk and the white part of the egg have to be taken out through that orifice.

The egg must be slightly warmed up in boiling water before making the orifice.

The disciple must paint the egg a blue color.

That empty shell must be placed next to our bed. The disciple will fall asleep while imagining to be inside, within the egg.

The Master Huiracocha says that in those instants one must invoke the God Harpocrates, by pronouncing the following mantra:

Har-po-crat-ist

Then, the God Harpocrates will carry the disciple within the egg. The disciple will feel a great itchiness or rash on his body.

The disciple will feel himself uncomfortable, because he will have that uncomfortable position with which the pigeon, while inside of an egg, is represented. However, the disciple must not complain, because the God Harpocrates will transport him to any far away place. The god will open the egg and will leave him there.

In the beginning, the student will only transport himself in his Astral Body. Later on the student will transport himself with his body in the Jinn State. This is a matter of much practice and tenacity.

The Jinn States permit us to perform all of these marvels. The Guru Litelantes showed me in a practical way how a physical body while in Jinn State can assume distinct forms, such as enlarging and shrinking itself by will.

Indeed, official science does not completely know about the physical body, but only about its purely primary or elementary aspects.

The scientists totally ignore that the physical body is plastic and elastic. Official anatomy and physiology are still in an embryonic state.

The forces that the Guru Litelantes taught me to command are the Harpocranian forces that boil and palpitate in the whole universe.

The **Har-po-crat-ist** forces are a variation of the Christic forces.

Wherever a Jinn State, an Astral projection, a temple in Jinn State, or an enchanted lake exists, the **Har-po-crat-ist** forces are found in an active function.

The disciple is accumulating these **Har-po-crat-ist** energies when he performs the practices of **Har-po-crat-ist**. Then, later on, these energies will truly allow him to perform marvels and prodigies.

I learned this marvelous science from the Guru Litelantes. She is my priestess-wife, who works in the superior worlds as one of the forty-two judges of Karma.

Mantra to Place the Physical Body in a Jinn State

The disciple who wants to travel with his physical body within the Astral Plane must enchant his body. The disciple must get sleepy by pronouncing the mantra:

To the little heaven, Philip

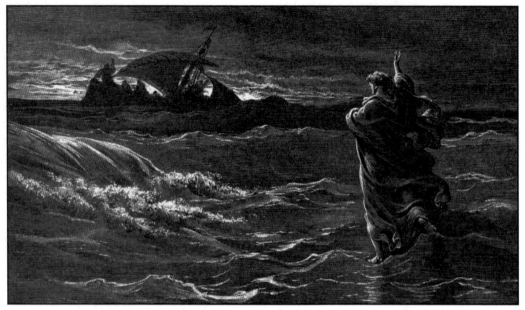

JESUS DEMONSTRATING THE POWER OF FAITH AND THE JINN STATES. ENGRAVING BY GUSTAVE DORÉ.

To the little heaven, Philip

To the little heaven, Philip

Then, he will leave his room and will direct himself in flesh and bones towards the house of his sick patients in order to medicate them. This is a type of voluntary somnambulism, a modification of somnambulism. What is needed is a lot of faith and tenacity until achieving success.

Another Jinn Practice

We, the Gnostics, can enter with flesh and bones into the other world any time we want to do so. Therefore, whosoever wants to enter into the other world in order to know and visit it with the body of flesh and bones, very well dressed with hat and fashionable shoes as when someone enters a garden party, then I give the clue:

1. Lie down on the side of your heart, with your head rested over the palm of your left hand.

2. You must become sleepy.

3. Reject from your imagination every type of dreaming and mental images.

4. Concentrate only and exclusively in the process of the dream.

5. When you feel that you are "asleep," then perform the following movements:

Sit on your bed. However, when you make this movement of sitting, do it with a lot of carefulness, in such a way that you will not awake. In other words, preserve your dreaming state, because the power is within the dream.

Stand on the floor with your feet, with the same carefulness of not awakening, because the power is within the dream.

Perform a little jump with the intention of floating in the other world.

If you do not float, then lie down and repeat the experiment again.

There are people who after having received this clue perform this experiment immediately. Yet, other people take weeks, months and even entire years in order to perform what others can do immediately after learning the clue. Everything depends upon the degree of evolution of every one. This is what is called in esotericism "Jinn State."

The powerful, energetic forces of the sub-consciousness are the ones that take the physical body out from the chemical-physical region and place it within the Astral Plane. This is how the physical body abandons the law of gravity and this chemical region in order to enter within the Astral Plane, where the laws of levitation reign.

As the smoke of the chimney is mixed with the atmosphere without confusion, in the same way these two worlds, Astral and physical, are mixed and they are inter-penetrated without confusion. Therefore, everything that I say can be confirmed by all those people who have the kindness of listening to me and have faith.

Nevertheless, I am sure that the thousands of readers from this twentieth century will mock these clues, because the people from this century only want to cohabit and get money, more money, and a lot more money. Therefore, this book is not for the barbarians of this twentieth century. This book is for the luminous humanity of Aquarius.

Those who perform this secret in order to enter with their physical bodies into the Astral Plane will transport themselves to the most far away places of the earth in a few seconds, because time and space do not exist within the Astral Plane. There, everything is an eternal "now," an eternal present.

The supra-sensible worlds are the celestial heavenly home of the Spirit.

Death is swallowed up in victory. O death where is thy sting? O grave, where is thy victory...? - Corinthians: 15:54-55

Esoteric Medication and Magical Works

Conjurations and Prayers

Royal Conjuration

I conjure all thy enemies, just as much thy internal as thy external ones, in the portal of Belen. I conjure them and I conjure them once again in case they have a pact with the devil, black magic, or backward creeds. I conjure them, so that they shall come humbly to thy feet, as the lamb of Christ reached the foot of the Cross. I conjure them, so that they shall come meekly, just as the lamb came from the cross to the eternal Father. With two I see them and with three I fasten them, in the name of the Father, the Son, and the Holy Spirit.

Explanation: 2 is Mother Nature and 3 is the three primary forces.

Prayer for Worms

Perjured animal, I conjure thee. Let all the worms drown in thy own blood, so that none will remain in thee.

Prayer of Our Lady Saint Martha for the Defense of the Body

O Saint Martha, thou art blessed, very beloved, and worthy of God, and thou walk on Mount Tabor. Thou entered and encountered the great serpent, then with the Mother of God's girdle thou tied and bound

it. Thus, thou bound the hearts of all my enemies who came against me in the name of the eternal Father and of the Holy Trinity.

Pronounce the "Apostle's Creed" three times.

For the Toothache

Saint Veronica was seated upon a stone. The Virgin passed and asked her, what's the matter with that fellow? He has a strong toothache and he cannot endure it. Remember the enduring breath and the cord that I gave thee, so that thou cannot suffer racking pain from any molar or any tooth. Amen, Jesus.

Pray "Hail, Mary" three times and "The Lord's Prayer" three times.

For Ringworm

Here I pray to the ringworm, from the very source where it starts and to where it ends in thy ribs. Ringworm, thou hast to disappear, ringworm. I believe in God, the Father.

Then, with a feather and writing ink, rub the affected area.

For the Evil Eye

Let the angels be with thee, in alliance in thy bed among the eleven thousand Virgins and one glory to Saint Anna.

Saint Anna begot Mary, Saint Isabel begot Saint John. With these seven words this evil will be healed.

To Defeat Demons

Thou who art the merciful and grandiose Virgin, I beseech thee, do not allow anything to fall on me. Let me be thy advocate.

To Combat the Demon

O Divine God! I want thou to help me to defeat this demon, that wherever I go thou shalt help me to defeat him. I want thou to protect me from any evil that comes against me. Save me from all evilness.

To Perform Massages to Heal without Pain

Jesus, Mary, and Joseph, most holy trinity, the three divine persons. Saint Blas ahead, Saint Peter behind. Saint Blas, if these words are good, then let the tendons and joints return to their place.

Apply these words in the name of Jesus Christ.

When Jesus Christ came to the world there were no injuries, no one maimed, no one lame, so let the injuries cease, and hail Mary.

Pray the "Apostle's Creed" three times. If the injury is not too severe, pray the "Apostle's Creed" three times. However, if the injury is very bad, pray the "Apostle's Creed" nine times. Rub menthol with salt onto the injury.

Prayer to the Aloe Plant

Cross, thou art holy and divine. Sorcerers and witches withdraw from this home. Such persons who intend to arrive here, let it be known that I am with God.

Sovereign God, set me free from treason and from ruination. Blessed be the most Holy Mary and the Consecrated Host.

Bless the Aloe with the sign of the cross.

The Magic Key

The magic key (iron key) must be magnetized with a lodestone. The magic key opens the doors from the past and gives access to the infernos.

The magic key makes disappeared objects and finds the treasures of the earth. Clearly, this key puts magic into action.

If this key is placed over an open Bible on any of the four gospels, then the key rotates and answers whatever is asked of it.

The gnomes must be invoked in order for the key to spin. The keys of ancient people are made of iron.

Prayer to the Gnomes

By the pole of lodestone that passes through the heart of the world, by the twelve stones of the holy city, by the seven metals that run inside the veins of the interior of the Earth, I conjure ye, subterranean workers, I call upon ye in the name of Christ and of GOB. Amen.

After reciting the above, ask for the object, money, or whatever has disappeared. Interrogate the subterranean workers. Thus, the key will spin. If the key does not spin, this is a result of a lack of faith. When one has faith, then one has power and the key spins. Any subconscious or infraconscious doubt, as insignificant as it might be, is enough in order for the key not to spin.

Method for asking: "Obey the Christ, subterranean workers. Tell me: is what I lost in this place? Or in this other place? Was it stolen by somebody? Etc."

If the key spins towards the right, then the answer is yes. If the key spins towards the left, then the answer is no.

The Magic Wand

Make for yourself a magic wand out of cedar wood, then pray the following magical words to the wand:

Elohim, Metraton, Adonai

Thus, the wand will become consecrated.

One operates magically with the magic wand. It serves in order to command the invisible forces of Nature, with the condition that we maintain upright behavior.

The forces of Nature will never obey one who is angry, lustful, greedy, envious, proud, lazy, gluttonous, jealous, resentful, evil, slanderous, etc.

Magic Mirror

Magic mirrors are very useful in practical magic. Write over your magic mirror the following mantric words:

Adam - Te - Dageram - Amrtet - Algar - Algas - Tinah

Always magnetize your mirror and use it in magic in order to clairvoyantly see whatever is necessary.

Keep your mirror sheltered or have it over your altar so that you can utilize it at any time that is necessary.

I advise you not to spy on the private lives of others or to calumniate people. Clairvoyance is developed with the condition of having very upright behavior.

Magic mirrors should never be missing from the Gnostic Lumisials. The hypersensitive people can see many marvels from the suprasensible worlds in such mirrors.

Magic Circle

When you trace around yourself a magic circle, whether it is with your sword, with your willpower and imagination united in vibrating harmony, or with both at the same time, you must pronounce the following mantras:

Helion, Melion, Tetragrammaton

The magician defends himself against attacks from the demons with the magic circle and the esoteric Pentagram.

Jinn States

If placing your body of flesh and bones within the fourth dimension is a very arduous task for you, if in spite of having done the effort you have not achieved it yet, then bathe yourself daily with aromatic herbs, and before falling asleep call the "seven potencies" so that they may assist in preparing your physical body.

Then, after your body is prepared, work again with the secrets that we have taught you in order to travel with your physical body through the fourth dimension.

One needs to have faith in the seven potencies. The seven potencies are not the seven spirits before the throne. They are seven masters who can prepare your body. *Ask and it shall be given to you, knock and it shall be opened to you.*

Astral Projections

If in spite of all the clues that we have taught in order to consciously travel in the Astral Body you have not achieved it yet, then do not feel discouraged. Study chapters sixteen to twenty-one of my book entitled *The Secret Doctrine of Anahuac.* [These chapters are included in the book *Dream Yoga* by Samael Aun Weor]. I promise you, beloved reader, that if you submit yourself to the discipline written in those cited chapters, then you will learn how to consciously travel through the Suprasensible Worlds. What is important is to perform everything correctly and to not dismay in your efforts. Then you will triumph.

Through this conversation that you and I are having via this book that you have in your hands, I sincerely tell you that the only thing that is of interest to me is that you progress. Truly, I want to help you.

To Defend Oneself from Lightning and from Fire

In order to defend oneself from lightning and fire, you must write upon the ceiling of your house and on the walls of the rooms of your house the following magical words:

Mentem, Santam, Spontaneum, Honorem, Deo, Patria, Liber

Against Danger from Bullets, Knives, Wounds, Enemies, Ambush, etc.

Are you in a dangerous situation? If so, filled with faith, recite the following words:

Fons Alpha Et Omega, Figa, Figalis Sabbaoth, Emmanuel, Adonai, O, Neray, Ela, Ihe, Reutone, Neger, Sahe, Pangeton, Commen, Agla, Matheus, Marcus, Lucas, Johannes, Titulus Triunphalis, Jesus Nazarenus Rex Iudaeorum, Ecce Dominicae Crucis Signum Fugite Partes Adversae, Vicit Leo De Tribu Judae, Radix David Alelluyah, Kyrie Eleison, Christe Eleison, Pater Noster, Ave Maria, Et Ne Vos, Et Venia Super Nos Salutare Tuum, Oremus.

(You must know all of these magical words by memory and you must pray them with faith in the moments of grave danger. Thus, you will save yourself from knives, bullets, secret enemies, ambush, etc., etc.).

Magic from the Memories of Nature

Do you want to see your past existences in a magic mirror? This is very simple. I am going to give you the following formula:

Place a lit candle to the right side of a mirror, in such a position that it will illuminate the mirror, yet without the mirror reflecting the image of the candle within it. You must turn off the rest of the lights within the room.

Do not think about anything. Breathe like newborn children breathe. Put the index, middle finger and your thumb of your right hand over your heart.

Pronounce the mantra **Om, Hum** with each palpitation of your heart. These words open the chakra of your heart where your past lives abide. Beseech your Divine

Mother to show you within the mirror your past lives. Ultimately, you will achieve it with patience.

The Secret Order of the Epoptae

Very ancient scriptures of Tibetan Tantra speak about a universal secret order from the Astral World that can initiate any aspirant during the normal, common, and current dream state, while out of the physical body.

It is emphatically stated that the powerful channels of force that emanate from the transcendental consciousness of the adepts of the Order of the Epoptae can be perceived in any part of the world.

The aspirant meets the adepts of this order during the sleep of his physical body.

In order to awaken the sacred fire, male initiates who do not have a wife and who march on the upright path can practice Sexual Magic with one of those females who soar up within the clouds. Such females are called "Dakinis."

Tibetan texts dedicate a considerable amount of space in order to praise and to disclose the beauty and grace of the Dakinis' form. They are represented with a beautiful contexture, ruby red skin, gentle and pensive faces, red eyes and red nails, and it is said that they exude the tenuous fragrance of a lotus bud.

Women who do not have a husband must not be preoccupied with this. In time, if they do not wed a husband, they will receive a deva from Nature as a husband and will practice Sexual Magic with him, in order to awaken their Kundalini or sacred fire, which always grants us magical powers.

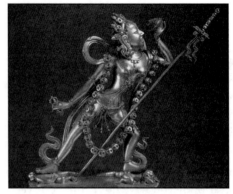

A DAIKINI

You must concentrate daily in the Master Tahuil, adept of the Order of the Epoptae. Thus, you will be assisted.

Go to sleep with your head facing towards the north. Relax your body, invoke Tahuil, and call upon the adepts of the Order of the Epoptae with the following prayer:

> *OM. I call, I invoke the Master Tahuil and the adepts of the Order of the Epoptae, so that they can take me out of my physical body and awaken me in the Astral World.*

The adepts from the Order of the Epoptae will educate you in the Astral World during the normal dream state.

When you awaken from your dream, practice a retrospective exercise in order to remember your astral experiences.

Sometimes, the Dakinis reincarnate as women of flesh and bones. Joyful is the man who can take one of those Dakini women as a spouse.

The Devas also reincarnate, and they too can serve as husbands for women who really want to follow the path of perfection.

Protection

Most Holy Mary, pious Mother, cover me with your mantle. Divine Cross, I ask Thee protection by these three names of Jesus, Joachin, and John.

Prayer of the Lodestone

O precious lodestone, you that ran along with the Samaritan woman, to whom you gave beauty and luck. I bring you gold for my treasure, silver for my house, copper so that I never lack but am always bountiful, coral so that in my house there will never befall envy or anything amoral. O Divine God, who gave to all men wisdom and power as the lodestone. May none of these powers be lacking within my house.

Prayer of Saint Paul (for the Snake)

Saint Paul said 'Jesus' when he put his foot upon the bolder. Saint Paul said 'Jesus' when he took his foot off of it. Saint Paul was so beloved by a so powerful God that he set me free from snakes and from poisonous animals. These words, which he uttered, I utter them because I know them, in the name of Jesus, Maryl and Joseph.

Pray one "Lord's Prayer" and three "Hail, Mary" prayers.

Jehovah God

In the name of Jehovah God, Christ Jesus, pray for my brethren, my father, my mother, my children, my nephews, my nieces, and all friends who are good hearted, by my glory to God, the Father, and the Holy Spirit.

To Enchant the Body

When you go to sleep, and while within the covers of your bed, pray the following prayer:

Philip, Philip, Philip, apostle of our Lord Jesus Christ, take me with my body.

To the little heaven, Philip. To the little heaven, Philip. To the little heaven, Philip. Amen.

Recite this magic prayer thousands of times and when you feel a great deal of drowsiness and a little bit of dreaminess, then get up from your bed while reciting the prayer. Jump immediately, fly and travel.

Astral Departures

DAILY EXERCISE: Any time that you are at your work, in the street, in your house, in the presence of a strange thing, or in front of a person whom you have not seen for a long time, ask yourself: "Am I in the Astral Body?"

Then, perform a small jump and if you float it is because you are within your Astral Body. Thus, you can fly and direct yourself to any place in the world. If you do not float, it is because you are within your body of flesh and bones.

When one practices this exercise during the day, then it is repeated during one's dreams and the result is that the consciousness awakens and experiences a lucid dream. One becomes aware that one is out of the physical body in the Astral World.

Serpents

There were seven islands in the Pacific Ocean that the ancient people called "Malabares." All sicknesses were healed there with serpents.

It was admirable to see the inhabitants of the Malabares islands skillfully handle many vipers.

Those people had a stature of three meters in height and their bones were elastic. They possessed double tongues, and their ears, which were divided by natural partitions, formed a double ear.

Those inhabitants of the Malabares islands could sequentially speak with two distinct persons in two distinct languages.

The Malabares disappeared overnight. Nobody knows what happened to those islands and their strange inhabitants.

The King of the World selected them. Now, they live with Him in "Agartha," the subterranean kingdom.

The inhabitants of the Malabares islands healed with serpents. For each sickness, they had a specific and defined serpent.

We already know that the rattlesnake serves in order to cure cancer. Rattlesnake meat is miraculous, yet the remedy is very jealous. It is enough for the sick person to consume any other remedy for the cancer in order for the rattlesnake remedy to become worthless.

I, myself, have cured several persons with cancer with the rattlesnake, and I am sure that ninety-nine percent of people with cancer can be cured with the rattlesnake, if they eat the rattlesnake meat until becoming healed.

To Conjure the Demons from the Possessed Ones

Burn before the possessed ones livers and hearts of fish, and recite with a lot of faith the Conjuration of the Seven of the Wise Solomon.

The possessed one must also be smudged with the smoke of sage and rue for nine days. These plants must be burned within charcoal embers.

To Drive the Snakes Away

Pronounce the following mantras:

Osi, Osoa, Asi

To Enchant the Snakes

Sing these magic words:

Osi, Osoa, Osias

Mantras to Become Invisible in Case of Danger

Have faith and pronounce the following magic words:

Athal, Bathel, Nothe, Jhoram, Asey, Cleyuhgit, Gabellin, Sameney, Mencheno, Bal, Labenentem, Nero, Meclap, Halateroy, Palcim, Tingimiel, Plegas, Peneme, Fruora, Heam, Ha, Ararna, Avora, Ayla, Seye, Peremies, Seney, Levesso, Hay, Barulachu, Acuth, Tural, Buchard, Caratim, Permisericordiam, Abibit Ergo Mortale, Perficiat Qua Hoc Opus, Ut Invisibiliter, Ire Possim. Amen.

Solar Conjuration to See Your Beloved One from a Distance

Take a blue paper, make an orifice in it, then filled with love and infinite faith, look at the rising Sun through that orifice while reciting the following dharani:

> *In the name of the holy and mysterious Tetragrammaton, with infinite humbleness, sincerely acknowledging that I am an infamous sinner, I conjure Thee, O Solar Spirit, by the eternal living God, so that Thou can console me by allowing me to see* (say the name of the beloved).
>
> *I do not intend to spy on her* (his) *life, neither to perform evil, but I only want to see her* (him) *with love.*
>
> *Anima Mea, Turbata Est Valde; Sed Tu Domine, Usquequo.*
>
> *Amen, Ra, Amen, Ra, Amen, Ra.*

Recite this prayer thousands of times, fixing your imagination and willpower and even your eyes on the King Star (Sun). At last, the beloved one will appear. You will see him or her, and you will have that great joy.

You will see the one whom you love, whether this one is your husband, son, daughter, boyfriend, girlfriend, etc.

Even if that person is dead, you will see him or her.

Magic Invocations

Invocation to Extinguish Blazing Fires

> *Hue Hueteotl, Hue Hueteotl, Hue Hueteotl, take the fire away. Extinguish this conflagration. Amen.*

Invocation to Unleash the Air with the Purpose of Taking the Fire Away or for Other Useful Goals - Barbas de Oro (Goldenbeard)

INVOCATION:

> *Barbas de Oro, Barbas de Oro, Barbas de Oro, blow. We need air. Amen.*

After reciting these words, you must whistle, so that Barbas de Oro (Goldenbeard), who is a Sylph from the air, will make the wind blow.

Invocation to Call the Undines from the Water

> *Veya, Vallala, Veyala, Helaya, Veya*

Sing these words when at the shore of rivers or seas and the Undines of the waters will come to your call.

Invocation to Make Rain

If there is a lack of rain and water is necessary, then pray the following:

> *Tlaloc, Tlaloc, Tlaloc, god of waters, bring the rain. We need water. We invoke thee in the name of our Lord Quetzalcoatl. Amen.*

Invocation to Invoke the Angels

Trace a circle on the ground over any place where two roads cross. Then, pronounce the Clavicle of Solomon and the name of the angel whom you want to call.

You must place yourself in the center of the circle. I advise you to perform this work on Good Friday at twelve midnight.

I suggest to you the idea of calling the Angel Adonai. That angel can become visible and tangible to your senses.

Do not be afraid. Speak with the invoked angel in tranquility.

Clavicle of Solomon

> *Per Adonai Elohim, Adonai Jehovah, Adonai Sabaoth, Metraton. On Agla, Adonai Mathom, Verbum Pitonicum Misterium Salamandrae, Conventum Silphorum, Antragnomorum Demonia Celi, Gad Almousin Gibor, Jeshua Evam Sariatniamic, Veni, Veni, Veni.*

INDICATION: The angels must be invoked with this clavicle.

Procedures for Magic Invocations

Since the air of the place where the angels are invoked must be prepared so that the invoked angels can become visible and tangible, it is convenient to know the names of the angels who govern the air during the distinct days of the week. Thus, we will prepare the magic air by invoking such genii.

Regents of the Air

Archan commands on Monday.
Samax commands on Tuesday.
Madiat, Vel, and **Modiat** command on Wednesday.
Guth commands on Thursday.
Sarabotes commands on Friday.
Maimon commands on Saturday.
Varcan commands on Sunday.

Instructions

FIRST: The sacred invocations must always be performed during the night.

SECOND: It is allowed or sanctioned to perform the angelic invocations only in order to ask for the healing of some gravely sick person or for some charitable work.

Whosoever invokes the angels for good and for the good of others marches in an upright manner.

THIRD: The angels can be invoked in any solitary spot in the mountains, where two roads merge and form a cross.

FOURTH: With the tip of a sword, trace a magic circle on the ground, around oneself.

FIFTH: The traced circle must be two meters in diameter and the invoker must place himself in the center.

SIXTH: Whosoever invokes the angels just because of dint of a game will not receive any type of answer.

SEVENTH: One must have a lot of faith, supreme concentration and meditation on the angel whom one wishes to invoke.

Perfumes for the Invocations

The perfumes for the invocations will be used in the place where the invocations will be performed.

It is clear that only the perfume of the day will be used.

Monday is governed by the Moon.
Tuesday is governed by Mars.
Wednesday is governed by Mercury.
Thursday is governed by Jupiter.
Friday is governed by Venus.
Saturday is governed by Saturn
Sunday is governed by the Sun.

The true order of the days of the week from the cosmic and magical point of view is the following:

After Saturday, which is the seventh day, follows Monday.

Monday, Wednesday, Friday, Sunday, Tuesday, Thursday, and Saturday. This is the authentic and legitimate cosmic order.

Perfumes

Saturn

The perfumes of Saturn, the ancient of the centuries, can and must be prepared with any type of aromatic roots and frankincense. It is also convenient to use branches of pine and cypress. Burn all of these mixed together at the location of the invocation.

Jupiter

The perfumes of Jupiter, the titan of heaven, can be prepared with scented fruits, with spices, such as clove and the very famous nutmeg.

Mars

The perfumes of Mars, the god of war, can be prepared with oak leaves, scented woods, sandalwood, and oleos.

Sun

The perfumes of the Sun are all types of gums, like frankincense, benzoin, and storax, as well as sunflower, flowers and leaves of laurel, etc.

Venus

The perfumes of Venus can be prepared with roses and violets.

Mercury

The perfumes of Mercury, the god of eloquence, can be conveniently prepared with all types of scented wood, aromatic seeds, cinnamon, cassia, nutmeg, cedar bark, etc.

Moon

The perfumes of the Moon must be prepared with eucalyptus, myrtle, asparagus, etc.

These perfumes will be used as smoke offerings by burning them within a small pan with charcoal embers at the location of the invocations.

People who are fearful, fornicating, adulterous and criminal, etc., must not perform these invocations.

Magic Exorcisms

After the magic circle has been traced and the air has been prepared by means of the perfumes, then the invoker (who is in the center of the circle) will recite the exorcism of that day (in which he is working) with great faith. Each day has its own exorcism.

Exorcism for Monday

With infinite humbleness and great love, in the name of the terrific Tetragrammaton, I invoke ye, ineffable beings.

In the name of Adonai and by Adonai, Adonai, Eye, Eye, Eye, Cados, Cados, Cados, Achim, Achim, Achim, La, La, La, strong La, thou, who always gloriously glows in the mountain of the Being, I beg thee for mercy. Help me now. Have pity on me, who has no value, who is nothing.

Adonai, Sabaoth, Amathai, Ya, Ya, Ya, Marinata, Abim, Ieia, creator of all that is and will be.

I beg thee in the name of all the Elohim who govern the first legion under the supreme command of Orfamiel and by the thirteen rays of the Moon and by Gabriel, so that thou can help me right now. I acknowledge that I am only a miserable slug from the mud of the earth. Amen.

Exorcism for Wednesday

I beg ye, divine Elohim, in the name of the sacred and terrific Tetragrammaton and by the ineffable names of Adonai Elohim, Sadai, Sadai, Sadai, Eye, Eye, Eye, Asamie, Asamie, Asamie, in the name of the angels of the second planetary legion, under the government of Raphael, Lord of Mercury, as well as by the holy name placed upon the forehead of Aaron, help me, assist me, come to my call. Amen.

Exorcism for Friday

Very humbly I beg ye, divine Elohim, by the mystical names On, Hey, Heya, ia, ie, Adonai, Saday, come to my call. I beseech ye, help in the name of the Tetragrammaton and by the sacred power of the angels of the third legion who are governed by Uriel, the regent of Venus, the star of dawn. Come Anael, come, come. I acknowledge my imperfections; yet, I adore thee and invoke thee. Amen.

Exorcism for Sunday

I, who am a wretched mortal, completely convinced of his (her) own nothingness and misery, dare to invoke the lions of fire and the blessed Michael.

By the Tetragrammaton I call now the fourth legion of angels of the Sun, hoping that Michael can have pity on me, Om, Tat, Sat, Tan, Pam, Paz, Amen.

Exorcism for Tuesday

I acknowledge what I am. Truly, I am a poor sinner who calls to and invokes the angels of Might, by means of the mantras: Ya, Ya, Ya, He, He, He, Va, Hy, Ha, Va, Va, Va, An, An, An, Aie, Aie, Aie, Ecl, Ai, Elohim, Elohim, Elohim, Tetragrammaton.

I invoke ye in the name of Elohim Gibor and by the regent of the planet Mars, Samael. Attend to my call.

Let the fifth legion of angels from the planet Mars assist me in the name of the venerable Angel Acimoy. Amen.

Exorcism for Thursday

Without pride, I acknowledge that I have no value, that I am nobody and that only my God has the power, wisdom, and love.

I beseech ye, ineffable devas, by the sacred names: Cados, Cados, Cados, Eschereie, Eschereie, Eschereie, Hatim, Hatim, Hatim, Ya, the corroborator of the centuries, Cantine, Jaym, Janic, Anie, Caibar, Sabaoth, Betifai, Alnaim and in the name of Elohim and Tetragrammaton and by the divine Zachariel who governs the planet Jupiter and the sixth legion of cosmic angels, attend to my call.

I beseech ye, ineffable beings, that ye assist me in this work. I beg ye by

the terrific Tetragrammaton, that ye help me here and now. Amen.

Exorcism for Saturday

Acknowledging my tremendous nothingness and interior misery, with complete humbleness, Casiel, Machatori, Sarakiel, attend to my call. I beseech ye, in the name of the holy and mysterious Tetragrammaton to come here.

Listen ye to me by Adonai, Adonai, Adonai, Eye, Eye, Eye, Acim, Acim, Acim, Cados, Cados, Cados, Ima, Ima, Ima, Saday; Io, Sar, Lord Orifiel, regent of the planet Saturn, chief of the seventh legion of ineffable angels.

Come, ineffable beings from Saturn. Come in the name of Orifiel and in the name of the powerful Elohim Casiel. I call upon ye, asking for help in the name of the Angel Booel, and by the star Saturn, and by its holy seals. Amen.

Invocations

When reciting the exorcism of the day, the invoker must place himself in the center of the circle, and must submerge himself in profound meditation, begging the planetary regent of that day to send him some of his holy angels.

While praying, meditating, and even weeping, the invoker must ask, supplicate, beseech. Faith must be intense and the supplication immense.

If there is not even a single atom of doubt within the invoker, the angel can become visible in the physical world. Any simple atom of doubt makes the magic phenomena of the materialization of any angel impossible.

The petition must be formulated with clarity and with a great deal of humility.

Fasting

Before performing the invocation, one must perform a fast for nine days. Pure water with honey (bee-honey) and lemon must be drunk during the fasting.

The invocation must be performed on the ninth day of fasting. Pure water sweetened with bee honey and some drops of lemon juice makes this fast possible.

The angels help in accordance with the Law and until permitted by the Law. The help that the angels grant us is processed in accordance with the Law, and never in accordance with our merely personal capriciousness.

When something is not granted to us, it is because we must pay what we owe. Instead of protesting, we must humbly incline ourselves before the verdict of the Law.

Planetary Regents

Gabriel is the regent of the Moon.

Raphael is the regent of Mercury.

Uriel is the regent of Venus.

Michael is the regent of the Sun.

Samael is the regent of Mars.

Zachariel is the regent of Jupiter.

Orifiel is the regent of Saturn.

Planetary Characteristics

Gabriel must be invoked on Monday.

Raphael must be invoked on Wednesday.

Uriel must be invoked on Friday.

Michael must be invoked on Sunday.

Samael must be invoked on Tuesday.

Zachariel must be invoked on Thursday.

Orifiel must be invoked on Saturday.

Indications

Our readers must not forget that the present day Saturday is the seventh day of the week and that the present day Sunday is the first day of the week according to the cosmic order (indicated on the former pages).

Thus, **Monday** is present day Sunday, **Wednesday** is present day Monday, **Friday** is present day Tuesday, **Sunday** is present day Wednesday, **Tuesday** is present day Thursday, **Thursday** is present day Friday and **Saturday** is present day Saturday.

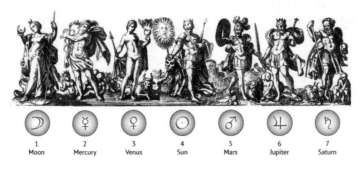

1	2	3	4	5	6	7
Moon	Mercury	Venus	Sun	Mars	Jupiter	Saturn

Planetary Specifications

Moon: Imagination, subconscious automatism, reproduction of species, travel, manual arts, practical arts, business related with liquid products, etc.

Mercury: Reasoning and rationalization, judicial disputes, civil matters, legal profession, science, everything that is related with the intellect, medical science, healing.

Venus: Artistic, creative imagination, dramas, comedies and tragedies, scenic art, love matters, conjugal problems, boyfriend and girlfriend matters, all that is related with the home and with children, etc.

Sun: Health, life, fertility, high dignitaries from the government, chiefs of companies, kings and lords of command, etc., etc.

Mars: Willpower, command, armies, wars, surgery, force and forces, events that imply struggles, etc., etc.

Jupiter: Wealth, poverty, favorable or unfavorable economical matters, laws, people's rights, high religious dignitaries, judges, matters related with the law, etc.

Saturn: The environment we live in, practical life, karma in action, the sword of justice that reaches us from heaven, real estate matters, lands, houses, properties, jail, death, etc.

Final Indications

The day of the invocation must be selected according to the problem we have.

The magic circle around the invoker must never be forgotten. As we have already stated, this circle must be traced on the ground with the tip of the sword.

The air must be prepared with the corresponding perfumes.

The regent of the air from the corresponding day must be invoked, in order to beg him to arrange the air so that the planetary genie or genii can become visible and tangible before us.

The planetary invocation must be performed when the mandatory prerequisites have been accomplished. The corresponding invocation of that day will be used for this purpose.

Any doubt, as insignificant as it might be, even when it is unconscious or merely subconscious, will make the invocation a failure.

Fearful people must abstain from performing these theurgic invocations, because they could fall down dead in the experiment.

These type of invocations are for very courageous people. The invocation must be repeated thousands of times until the invoked genie becomes present.

Whosoever performs invocations for revengeful purposes, for a desired vengeance, for egotistical reasons, with envy, etc., will fail. They will not achieve anything with the invocation.

Theurgy is only possible based upon a lot of patience. Whosoever does not achieve the triumph in the first experiment must repeat the experiment thousands of times until triumphing.

Iamblicus was a great theurgist who worked with the planetary genii. It is obvious that this great master possessed faculties attained by great super-efforts and sacrifices. The theurgic faculties of Iamblicus were extraordinary.

Matrimonial Future

Single Gnostic women can explore their future in order to learn about their matrimonial possibilities. This is not a crime.

Magical Procedure

In your bedroom, establish two identical mirrors according to the binary of man and woman. A lit candle must be placed in front of each mirror.

The two mirrors must be positioned face to face. Each one will have its own lit candle, yet placed in such a way that the lit flame is reflected within the glass. The candles must be made out of wax.

Then, the woman must sit and with a loud voice sing the following magical words three times:

Kto, Enoy, Sonnjoy, Kto, Moy, Viajnoy, Tot, Pokajetsia Ninie

After pronouncing these mantras, dharani, or words of power, the woman must direct her sight with fixed intensity towards either of the two mirrors, intelligently choosing the most distant and obscure space where the magical apparition will appear.

It is advisable to pray the "Pater Noster," which is "The Lord's Prayer," before performing the experiment. Thus, in this way, by asking permission of our Father, who is in secret, is how the help of the Father will be received and the future husband will appear within the mirror.

The magical words *"Lucia, Stof, Lub, Salem, Sadil"* can and must also be recited during this magic experiment. This experiment must be performed at twelve midnight.

The Magic Mirror

The mirror of high magic is esoterically prepared in forty-eight days. The esoteric work is begun during the new moon and is concluded during the following full moon.

Success is attained with permission of the Father who is in secret. Truly, the Father of all the lights is the one who commands. If we want to work uprightly and with true dignity in White Magic, then we must start any esoteric work by begging the Father, asking permission of the Father who is in secret. This is how we will not fall into mistakes.

All things that are interesting to us can be seen within the magic mirror if the Father gives permission, if He helps, if He wants.

If the proper preparation of the magic mirror is what is wanted, then one must live in sanctity and total chastity during the time of its preparation.

It is necessary to dedicate oneself to performing charitable works during the whole of that time.

Acquire a very gleaming sheet of steel, very well polished. Write upon this sheet, near its four edges, the following magical words in a successive order: **Jehovah, Elohim, Metraton, Adonai.**

Each word must be written on the endmost part of each side. Thus, the four words will be distributed upon the furthermost parts of the four sides.

Devoutly place the steel sheet on top of a white and very beautiful cloth. In this way, you will present the gleaming sheet of steel before the rays of the moon while reciting the following prayer:

O Father of mine, O Isis,
Divine Mother, Saidic Mother,
Tetragrammaton, Tetragrammaton,
Tetragrammaton. Prepare for me
this mirror. Grant me the power to
look into it, and ask the resplendent
Angel Azrael to have the kindness of
appearing within this mirror.

Azrael, Azrael, Azrael, I adore
thee and I invoke thee. Come in
the name of the Tetragrammaton,
Amen, Amen, Amen.

Once this magic invocation is performed, branches of laurel must be burned in order to impregnate the magic mirror with the smoke of the branches.

After, the mirror will be perfumed with roses and violets, which will be thrown over the magic mirror.

Finally, and in order to conclude with this work, the following invocation must be recited with a lot of faith.

Invocation

In this, by this and with this mir-
ror of the Tetragrammaton, by
the Tetragrammaton and in the
Tetragrammaton, I implore the mys-
terious help of the Angel Azrael.

Once this invocation is completed, the mirror must be perfumed with the smoke of frankincense and myrrh. Then, one will blow on the mirror three times and with intense faith one must recite the following words:

Do not abandon me Azrael, I know
that I am a miserable slug from the
mud of the world.

I know that I am a poor sinner. I
know that I am walking on the path
of evil. All of this I know, yet I love
Thee, Azrael. I ask Thee so that
Thou can help me. Azrael, I implore

help from Thee. Azrael, come to me
in the magic and esoteric name of
Falma, by Falma, in Falma. Come
to this mirror Azrael, come, come,
come.

To conclude, one has to place the right hand over the mirror while beseeching the Father to send Azrael.

This has to be performed for forty-eight nights, until the Angel Azrael appears in the mirror. The Angel Azrael will appear in the shape of a beautiful child.

When the angel appears, then one has to beg him, so that he can always assist us when we work with the mirror.

Indications about the Magic Mirror

When the Angel Azrael appears in the mirror, then it is the sign that the mirror is already prepared. If in spite of all this the Angel Azrael does not appear, then you must be resigned that you cannot work with the mirror.

The Angel Azrael will not appear if we are unworthy. All the doors are closed for the unworthy, but one: the door of repentance.

Whosoever attains triumph with the Angel Azrael must only work in secret, without saying anything to anybody. The sacred, blessed mirror that was blessed by the Angel Azrael must remain in secrecy.

Whosoever divulges their works with the magic mirror, whosoever utilizes the magic mirror in order to spy on private lives, will lose the granted grace of the Angel Azrael.

The mirror must be utilized in order to consult about sacred matters. Each time that one works with the Angel Azrael, one must invoke the Angel with much respect and faith.

The Angel Azrael is a perfect creature. The Angel Azrael is the one who has the power of making us see the longed for answers within the mirror.

Therefore, this is why we must always ask for the help of the Angel Azrael during the works with the magic mirror.

The Magic Key of Pacts

By means of the magic key of the pacts of mystery, one can make the invoked genii appear.

This signifies that during the invocations of the holy theurgy, the magic key must be grasped in the moments of praying in order to beseech the presence of the ineffable gods.

This key or Solomonic clavicle is certainly the "dominatur" of the "sanctum regnum."

That key symbolizes the very same keys of the kingdom, or the key of the ark of science.

The key must be prepared on a legitimate Sunday, at the precise moment of sunrise. The key must be made with gold, brass, and bronze.

In order to make this magical amulet, the first hour of the King Star (the Sun, sunrise) must be chosen. Precisely, this should be on the authentic Sunday, in accordance with the cosmic order, which is: Monday, Wednesday, Friday, Sunday, Tuesday, Thursday, and Saturday. We already know that the present Saturday is cosmically correct and that after Saturday follows Monday.

In the moment of preparation, a small piece of lodestone must be added to the magic key of pacts and the following magical prayer must be recited:

Prayer

By the holy and mysterious Tetragrammaton; by the grace granted with the Elohim of the Light; by the Father of all the lights; by the power that the Ancient of Days grants to those who love him; by the power granted to the seven planetary regents; by the power of the ineffable beings: Adonai, Elochais, Almanab, to whom I beg for help:

Let this key remain authorized by the Gods in order to call upon the ineffable ones. Amen.

Every morning on Sundays, at the rising of the King Star (sunrise), seven grams of wheat must be put inside of the bag where the magic key is carried, as an offering to the seven planetary genii.

Also, little pieces of steel filings must be put inside the bag, as nourishment for this magical amulet.

When placing it over the heart, the following prayer must be prayed:

O King Star! Christ Sun, help me in the name of the holy and mysterious Tetragrammaton. Prepare for me this clavicle, so that when I show it to the angels, they can answer my call. Amen.

Esotericism of the Laurel

We must chew laurel leaves while we are submerged in profound meditation for long hours. This is how we can see the things that will occur in the future. Unquestionably, it is known that dried laurel has the magical virtue of prognosticating for whoever is questioning it whether something that is waited for will be prosperous or unpleasant.

If one laurel branch tossed on to flames is burned without producing the least bit of noise, then the outcome will be terrible.

On the contrary, if the branch of dried laurel is burned with great noise, intensely crackling and sparking, then it is announcing a total success.

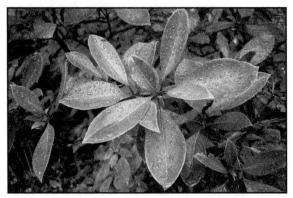

LAUREL

Divination through Fire

If you want to foretell through magical methods something that will occur to you, something that you are awaiting, some befalling event, then buy three green candles. If you do not find them with that color in the market, then paint them with green paint.

Place these three candles in three separated candle holders or candlesticks and form a triangle with them. Light each one of the three candles.

Once this is made and the candles are lit by means of some flammable object that must not contain sulphur, with all of your love you will call the six principal chiefs of the salamanders of fire.

You will pronounce the names of these six chiefs:

Vehniah, Achajad, Jesabel, Jeliel, Cathethel, Mehahel

When the candles are lit, you must not take from them even the smallest piece of their tinder or wick.

Once the magical invocation is made to the six chiefs of the salamanders, then you must carefully observe the actions of each flame. If the flames of the candles oscillate from left to right, then this announces some extraordinary event.

If the flames oscillate in the form of spirals, then you can be sure that there are many intrigues from your enemies. If the fire disappears, then some treason against you exists, or treason against the person or persons who have come to consult you.

If the resplendence of the fire increases and also happily crackles, then this is an announcement of total triumph, of formidable success.

Before performing this magical experiment, pray very slowly and meditate on "The Lord's Prayer." Ask permission of your Father, who is in secret, in order to perform this experiment.

Invocation of the King of the East

The King of the East will be invoked within a magic circle that will be traced on the ground. This circle will be two or three meters in diameter in any place in the mountains where two roads intersect and form a cross. The invocation must be performed at twelve midnight. The invoker will place himself in the center of the circle and will have his face and body directed towards the east. Then, the following invocation must be recited:

Prayer

Acknowledging that I am a monster of evil, a vile slug from the mud of the earth who has no value, knowing that I am a poor sinner, I invoke the powerful Lord Magoa, king of the east of the world. I call him in the name of the sacred Tetragrammaton. I conjure by the Tetragrammaton. I call by the holy and mysterious Tetragrammaton. I weep humbly asking thee, so that thou can answer this call.

In the name of thy Father, who is in secret, and of thy Divine Mother Kundalini, come to me, powerful king. Enter thee into the physical world, make thyself visible and tangible before me. In the case that thou cannot assist to this humble call due to thy cosmic works, then I beg thee, powerful lord, to send me Madel, and if this is not possible either, then the Genii Massayel, Asiel, Satiel, Arduel, Acorb, who obey thee, can come to me.

I know that thou, powerful lord of the east, can help me in accordance with justice and mercy. Amen, Amen, Amen.

Once the invocation is finished, then the invoker will then sit in the middle of the circle, meditating on the king of the east, weeping, acknowledging that he is a poor sinner, and repeating the prayer with his mind and heart, until the physical body becomes sleepy.

If the invoker performs this work correctly, then he will be assisted by the king of the east or by the genii who are sent by him. One must not be afraid in the presence of these divine beings.

When the lord of the east or his genii become visible, then ask whatever you wish. It is written: *"Knock and it shall be opened unto you, Ask and it shall be given you."*

We must not forget, by any means, that everything will be done in accordance with the Law. Everything will be arranged for us not in the way that we want, but as the Law wants. Thus, we must humbly bow before the verdict of the Law.

Invocation of the King of the South

O, Egym! Powerful lord of the regions of the south, most worthy master: with complete humbleness, acknowledging the interior misery in which I find myself, and with great love, i call thee and invoke thee. I am not worthy to call upon thee, yet i love thee. I beg to thee by the holy and mysterious Tetragrammaton. Come unto me, great king, I beseech thee. However, I know, oh lord, that thy labors are very great. Therefore, in case that thou art very occupied, then I very humbly prostrate myself before thee and I beg thee to send unto me the genie Fadal or the other divine genie named Nastrache.

Grant me this, oh powerful lord. I beseech this unto thee in the name of thy Father who is in secret, and of thy Divine Mother Kundalini. Amen, Amen, Amen.

Indications

This invocation will be performed in the center of the magic circle and with the face towards the south. Once this invocation is recited, the invoker will seat himself in the center of the circle.

Once seated, the invoker will meditate on the content of each word and will acknowledge his own nothingness and interior misery. He will greatly weep while calling the king of the south.

When the king or his genii will present themselves, then with humbleness one must ask for whatever is wished. *"Knock and it shall be opened unto you, Ask and it shall be given you."* Everything will be granted to us, yet not as we want, but as the Law wants.

Invocation of the King of the West

Powerful King Bayemon, who wisely governs the western regions of the planet Earth, listen to me, oh great lord.

Humbly, prostrated at thy feet, I invoke thee in the name of the holy and mysterious Tetragrammaton. Divine lord, have pity on me because I am a sinner.

I know that I have no value, because I am a miserable slug from the mud of the earth. Yet, I call upon thee, oh lord, in the name of thy Father who is in secret, and of thy Divine Mother Kundalini. Come, oh lord. Attend to my call by the Christ and by the Tetragrammaton.

In case that thou art very occupied in thy cosmic works, then send unto me the Genie Passiel Rosus. As I, myself, am nothing, as I have no value, I beg thee to forgive my boldness when I invoke thee. Bless me, oh lord, and become visible and

tangible before me. Amen, Amen, Amen.

The invoker will seat himself in the center of the circle traced on the ground in the place that we have already mentioned, which is in the mountains at the crossing of two roads.

The invoker will meditate on the king of the west, and when he appears, then he must ask what is wished for. It is necessary to have humility and to incline before the verdict of the Law. Everything will be done not as the invoker wants it, but as the Law wants. The invocations must always be performed at midnight in the mountains and with a lot of humility.

Invocation of the King of the North

Oh thou divine and ineffable Amaimon! Solar king of the north, humbly and with acknowledgment that I am an infamous sinner, I invoke thee in the name of thy Father who is in secret, and by thy Innermost Christ and by thy Holy Spirit and by thy Divine Mother Kundalini.

Listen to my plea, oh powerful lord. Come unto me in the name of the Tetragrammaton. If thy cosmic labors do not allow thee to assist me in these moments, then send me by the holy and mysterious Tetragrammaton the divine genii Madael, Laaval, Bamulahe, Belem, Ramat, or any of the genii who are under thy direction and government, all of them revested in a beautiful human form.

In the name of the holy and mysterious Tetragrammaton, humbly I beseech thy assistance. In the name of my interior God and of my Divine Mother Kundalini and by Sechiel, Barachiel, Balandier, as Beings, come unto me. Do not abandon me, oh powerful lord. Tetragrammaton, Tetragrammaton, Tetragrammaton. Amen, Amen, Amen.

As we already have stated, the invocations must be performed in the mountains where two roads cross, at twelve midnight.

The magic circle must be traced on the ground with the tip of the sword. The invoker, standing in the center of the circle, with his face towards the north, will invoke the king of the north.

Once the invocation is performed, the invoker must sit on the ground, in the center of the circle, meditating on the king of the north, until this king appears. Then the petition will be humbly done.

We must bow before the verdict of the Law. Fearful people must abstain themselves from making these invocations, because they can die of terror. Cardiacs must not perform these invocations either, because they can fall dead instantaneously.

Magic Secret to Travel Through the Airs of Mystery

The male or female magician must remain lying down for three days on their bed, without eating anything, nourishing themselves only with water, within which will be poured some drops of lemon juice and very pure honey (bee honey).

The head of the bed must be situated towards the north. The magician must meditate on Philip, the great apostle of Jesus Christ, during those three days.

The magician will also pray the "Pater Noster," which is "The Lord's Prayer," profoundly meditating on the meaning of each word from this most holy prayer that was taught by the Adorable One.

The magician will ask permission of the Father in order to travel with his physical body in a Jinn State through the Astral space of the universe. He or she will beseech the help and assistance of Philip. Once the three days have passed, then the magician can get up from the bed. The bed must then be cleaned and arranged with clean sheets, pillows, blankets, and clean bedspreads.

The room, sleeping compartment, or bedroom must be perfumed, swept, and washed very well.

Not a single piece of clothing should be hung on the ceiling or on the walls, because that damages the experiment.

Upon the day in which the magician gets up, he must continue nourishing himself with water within which is mixed honey (bee honey) and some drops of lemon juice.

At night, after a dinner based on fruit and water (prepared in the already indicated manner), the male or female magician will very secretly direct themselves towards their bedroom. Then, seven candles must be lit. The seven candles must be placed on a seven-armed candelabrum (or on seven candlesticks, or on two candelabras of three arms each, plus one candlestick for a single candle).

Subsequently, a very clean mantle must be placed over a table inside the bedroom. The table must be round, with three legs.

Three loaves of bread, which must be blended with barley flour, and three glasses of fresh and crystalline water must be placed on the table.

Then, very slowly and meditating, the magician will recite with the mind and with the heart filled with faith, the following magical prayer:

Prayer

Besticirum cosolatio, veni, ad me, vertu, creon, creon, o creon, cartor, laudem, omnipotentis et, nom, commentor, star, superiur, carta, bient, laudem, om, viestra, principien, da, montem, et, inimicos, meos, o, prostantis, vobis, et, mihi, dantes, quo passium, fieri, sui, cisibilis. Amen, Amen, Amen.

The male or female magician must recite this prayer thousands of times while ever so slightly becoming sleepy.

Finally, three mysterious ladies or three magical gentlemen will arrive. This matter pertains to three Jinn persons from the fourth or fifth dimension.

It is clear that three ladies will arrive if the invoker is a male, yet if it is a female magician, a woman who calls and prays, then three elegant Jinn gentlemen from the world of mystery will arrive.

Unquestionably, these three persons will utilize the Tarot and will cast their lot in order to define positions and to know who among them will be the one who will assist us and take us to wherever we wish.

These persons will drink and eat; they will converse amongst themselves. Then, the best will come.

After all of this, the magical person who has to help us will approach us. We must beg this person to carry us with our physical body to any place of the earth.

If they tell us or command us to get up, it is necessary to obey.

When the body is felt with that state of lassitude as when one goes to sleep, then in that state is where one senses the invoked genii.

We must get up from the bed in that state. The genii will assist us.

The Jinn person who will be in charge of us will take us to the place that we will indicate. The physical body delectably floats while inside of the magical regions of the earth. Thus, this is how we can transport ourselves to any place of the earth.

Indications

The previous Latin prayer must be learned by memory with the goal of correctly working with this secret, which serves in order to travel through the superior dimensions of Nature.

Faith is the foundation of this magical work. Without faith, one fails with this experiment. If the invoker is afraid, then he must not perform this work.

Thus, the Gnostic medics can travel with their physical bodies within the fourth vertical in order to assist their patients.

Each time that the Latin prayer is recited, then one will beseech by saying: *"Assist me genii, assist me, take me with my body."* This phrase must be repeated, filled with faith, between prayer and prayer.

Thus, one triumphs. This science is for the people with faith. One needs to know how to be serene, one needs to know how to be patient.

If someone does not triumph with the first experiment, it is because his mind is degenerated.

Then, he or she must repeat thousands, millions of times the experiment until triumphing.

Magic from the Woodlands

In the woodlands, in the mountains and villages, there are certain magical prayers that are very simple, yet of tremendous power.

Many times we have become overwhelmed over certain extraordinary magical events. Then, when we investigated, we discovered the formulae of those magical events. Those formulae stand out because of their simplicity.

Obviously, those who use such formulae are people who are extraordinarily simple and filled with a terrific and frightening faith.

Once upon a time (it does not matter when), a certain worker from the Summum Supremum Sanctuarium from the Sierra Nevada was gravely wounded on his foot. Immediately and filled with faith, I recited for him a magical prayer that instantaneously stopped the hemorrhage that was coming out of his wound.

This prayer is the following:

Prayer
With the blood of Adam, death was born; with the blood of Christ, life was born. Oh blood, stop flowing out!

Jinn Marvels: Nahualism

People who are very civilized, who always laugh at the magic of the woodlands, sometimes pass through very tremendous surprises.

I knew the case of a "nahual" who knew how to transport himself to remote distances while in a Jinn state, through the fourth dimension.

The formula was extremely simple: that man, filled with faith and without admitting a single atom of doubt into his mind, walked on his hands and feet, while imitating a mule with his imagination and willpower. Then, while walking around the whole patio of his house, he recited the following magical prayer:

Here is where the lame mule has passed through; here is where it has passed through, through here, through here.

That nahual believed himself to be a mule; he had no doubts about it; he was inebriated with that image while reciting that prayer.

Undoubtedly, the moment in which he submerged himself within the fourth dimension always arrived. He took on an animalistic form. This is not unusual among the nahual people. Even when the modern scientists deny these types of magical incidents, it does not matter, because by no means will the "nahual" people and "nahualism" cease to exist.

Nahualism

If medical science truly knew about the human body, then it would never doubt the "nahual" people, nor would they doubt the famous "nahualism," which is the magic of the woodlands.

When submerged within the fourth dimension, a physical body can change its shape. When submerged within the superior dimensions of Nature, a physical body can float in space.

If a nahual wants to assume the shape of an eagle, then it is enough for him to recite this magical prayer:

Prayer
Here is where the flying eagle has passed through; here is where it

has passed through, through here, through here.

It is obvious that imagination and willpower, united in a vibrating harmony, accompanied with action and immense faith, permits the "nahual" person to put his physical body inside the superior dimensions of Nature.

Thus, by means of action, imagination, and willpower harmoniously united the physical body can take the shape of the eagle. Then, one can really fly like an eagle.

When we say action, imagination, and willpower harmoniously united, we must be clearly comprehended.

If we are going to take the shape of an eagle, then we must imagine that our arms are the wings and that our feet and legs are eagle's feet and legs, and that the whole of our body is an eagle's body. Thus, with the imagination and willpower united in a vibrating harmony, filling ourselves with a frightful and immense faith, we will walk inside of our room moving the wings or arms, being absolutely sure that we are eagles, while pronouncing the prayer: *"Here is where the flying eagle has passed through, here is where it has passed through, through here, through here."*

It is obvious that imagination and willpower, united in a vibrating harmony, and when accompanied with actions, produce astral inebriation. Then, the physical body, tremendously saturated with imponderable fluid, really takes on the shape of the eagle.

When reaching this point of high magic, the physical body enters into the fourth vertical. If we toss ourselves into fearless flight, then we can travel upon the clouds to any place of the world.

The white nahual must never be preoccupied with the return, which is performed quite normally when one wishes to do so.

The magical formula that we have taught can be used to take the shape of any other animal. For example: if the nahual wants to take the shape of a white dove, then he will utilize the magical formula by saying:

Here is where the flying dove has passed through; here is where it has passed through, through here, through here.

Once this is said, then that shape will be intentionally taken by means of imagination and willpower united in a vibrating harmony, without forgetting the practical action.

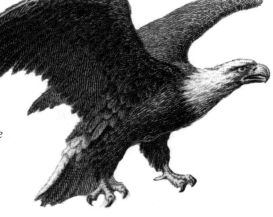

Much has been written in these times about esoteric matters. Yet, it is truly lamentable that the aspirants do not know about White Nahualism.

We, the Gnostics, are eminently practical. We do not like to waste our time miserably. We want our disciples to travel with their physical bodies within the superior dimensions of Nature.

When we want to take the shape of any animal, it is convenient to get up from our beds in the instant of being sleepy. Then, by walking inside of our room, whether in a shape of an eagle, whether in a shape of a white dove, whether in a shape of a sheep or lion, etc., we must work with the magical formula as indicated in this chapter.

The dream has to be kept as a precious treasure, by being careful of not losing it in the instant of getting up from our bed, in order to make the experiment.

Every Gnostic medic must learn to travel with his physical body in a Jinn state, in order to assist his patients from a distance.

The Angel Anael likes to convert himself into an innocent dove, in order to travel through the space of mystery.

The Buddhas of Compassion enjoy taking the marvelous shape of the lions of the Law, and this is not a crime.

Elementotherapy

Medicinal Plants

Anti-rheumatic Plants

Ash tree (leaves): use as an infusion; use for rubbing; and use for fumigation (burning).

Lemon: use the juice for rubbing and drink the juice in water without sugar.

Sweet Basil: use as an infusion; use for rubbing; and use for fumigation.

Wormwood: use as an infusion; use for rubbing; and use for fumigation.

Sage: use as an infusion; use for rubbing; and use for fumigation.

Rosemary: use as an infusion; use for rubbing; and use for fumigation.

Elder: use as an infusion; use for rubbing; and use for fumigation.

Each one of these plants cure articular and muscular rheumatism. They clean the skin of bad fluids, etc.

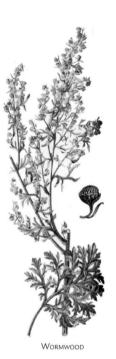

WORMWOOD

Anti-nervous and Calmative Plants

Red poppy (flowers, *Papaver rhoeas L.*), orange leaves, tincture of valerian, and linden tree leaves are anti-nervous and calmative plants.

Any of these plants can be taken as an ordinary beverage in order to calm the nerves and to dispel headaches.

Each one of these plants is the physical body of an elemental creature of Nature. If you want to succeed in healing sicknesses by utilizing curative plants, then there is the need to bless the plant and to command the vegetal elemental to cure the sick person. Again, I repeat, the plants are not the ones that cure; it is the vegetal elementals or the vital principles that are hidden within each herb, root and tree that cure.

This science of elementotherapy is solidly based upon the medical wisdom of the master of the White Lodge, Paracelsus.

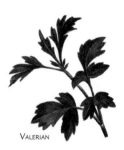

VALERIAN

Therefore, all of those students of Spiritualism, Theosophy, and the Rosicrucian Order who criticize elementotherapy are totally ignorant of this profound branch, which the illustrious Master Paracelsus granted to us.

Depurating Plants

Sarsaparilla (*smilax officinalis*), "gualanday" (*jacaranda spp.*), Grass, ash tree (leaves), walnut tree (leaves), horsetail (the whole plant, *equisetum arvense l.*), Maguey (root, *agave americana l.*), "Martin galvis" (flowers and leaves) are purifying plants.

Each one of these plants has the following properties: expels away venomous substances from the blood; cures chronic head colds, old rheum, gout, rheumatism, lithiasis, white discharge, discharge from the urethra, venereal sicknesses, syphilis, gonorrhea, rashes, scrofula, sicknesses of the skin, fistulas, sicknesses of the kidneys, eczema; and in general expels bad fluids from the blood.

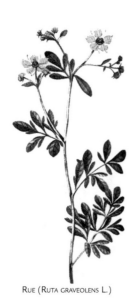

HORSETAIL (*EQUISETUM ARVENSE L.*)

Diuretic Plants

Lemon (juice), horsetail (the whole plant, *equisetum arvense l.*), Pellitory-of-the-wall (*parietaria diffusa* or *p.Officinalis*), licorice, grass, avocado tree (its tender leaves), medlar (seeds), pine (cones), cañaigre (*rumex hymenosepalus torr.*), elder (flowers and leaves), sarsaparilla (roots, *smilax officinalis*), cane (root), "caracola" (*besleria spp;* the part that looks like little eggs) are diuretic plants.

Each one of these plants serves against dropsy, gout, lithiasis, illness of the kidneys, urinary irritation, cold of the bladder, retention of the urine, etc.

Emmenagogue Plants

Wormwood (leaves, *artemisia absinthium l.*), celery (seeds), mugwort (leaves, *artemisia vulgaris l.*), chamomile (flowers), feverfew (flowers, *chrysanthemum parthenium l.*), rue (*ruta graveolens l.*), fennel (seeds and leaves) are emmenagogue plants.

Any of these plants serve in order to bring on menstruation, to regulate its normal activity, to regulate suppressed, tardy or heavy menstruation, to fortify the organs, to tone the woman's nervous system, to combat neuralgia, nervous vomiting, etc.

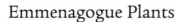

RUE (*RUTA GRAVEOLENS L.*)

Febrifuge Plants

Chiquichiqui (orimaco), borage, chuquiragua, cuacia, zarpoleta, eucalyptus (leaves), quinoa (cortex), ash (powdered cortex), cedrón (seeds), canagre, guaco, orange leaves, rosemary.

These plants can be taken by infusion, decoction or maceration in order to cut the fever and to impede the reappearance of eruptive, ardent and bilious fevers.

Laxative Plants

Almond oil, castor or resin oil, senna leaves, rhubarb in powder, are laxatives.

Restorative Plants

Wormwood (flowers and shoots, *artemisia absinthium l.*), chamomile (flowers), cinchona (bark, *cinchona spp.*), coca (leaves, *erythroxylon spp.*), fennel (seeds), lemon balm (leaves, *melissa officinalis l.*), and parsley are restorative plants.

They can be consumed in a decoction, infusion or maceration. Any of these plants have the power to stimulate and increase the vital forces of the organism.

Vermifuge Plants

In order to eject intestinal parasites

Garlic (cloves), pumpkin seeds in sugared water, lemon juice in sugared water on an empty stomach, etc., can be used.

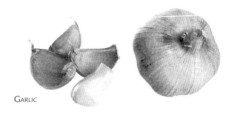

Garlic

Zodiacal Plants

The plants of **Aries** are similar to the head of the human being, and they belong to the element fire.

The plants of **Taurus** are similar to the human neck, and they belong to the element earth.

The plants of **Gemini** are similar to the arms, hands, and back of the human being, and they belong to the element air.

The plants of **Cancer** have in their leaves the form of the liver or spleen. They show spots, and show five petals in their flowers. They belong to the element water.

The plants of **Leo** have the shape of the heart in their fruits as well as in their leaves, and they belong to the element fire.

The plants of **Virgo** are similar to the stomach and intestines, and they belong to the sign of earth.

The plants of **Libra** are hot, humid, and aerial. They are similar to the kidneys, bladder, and the navel.

The plants of **Scorpio** are similar to the genitals, and they have an offensive odor. They are hot and humid.

The plants of **Sagittarius** belong to the element fire, and they are similar to the buttocks.

The plants of **Capricorn** are cold and dry; they have greenish flowers and a skeletal figure, similar to the knees.

The plants of **Aquarius** are similar to the calves, and they are aerial.

The plants of **Pisces** belong to the element water, and they look like the feet and toes.

Each of these plants serves the organ that it is similar to. Thus, the leaves that have the shape of a heart serve for the heart, the plants similar to a snake serve for what the shape shows. Mother Nature is very sapient; yet, the human being is eager to ignore her. The human being has become arrogant, and so he ignorantly wants to transcend Mother Nature.

An authentic index of astrological plants must be structured upon this base of stellar analogies, since truly (it is sad to say), it is painful to see how many authors attribute to one zodiacal sign the same plant that other authors attribute to a different zodiacal sign. Therefore, all that is written about astrological botany is totally wrong.

The Gnostic medics must return into the bosom of the blessed Goddess Mother of the world, in order to investigate on their own account within the great laboratory of Nature.

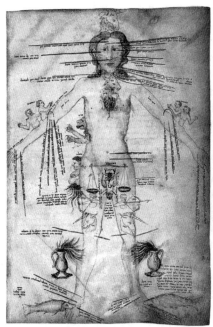

Hebrew manuscript, 14th century.

Plants and their Planetary Influence

Lunar Plants

The plants that belong to the moon are insipid. They always live in or near water, and are cold and milky. Commonly, they have big leaves. These plants have varied sizes with white flowers that have a very delicate smell. Eucalyptus is a lunar tree.

The lunar plants and trees are the physical bodies of the lunar elementals. The Arhuaco Mamas named the Moon "La Saga Tima."

The lunar elementals are the elementals of the water. Some Chinese adept artists and some Buddhist priests have painted them in beautiful paintings.

The great elemental kings of the water can make the student remember those remote epochs of Arcadia in which the human being worshipped Mother Nature. They offered her the first fruits of their harvest as an act of thanksgiving to the gods of the water, who watered the earth with beneficial rain.

These elementals of the water are known by the names of nymphs, nereids, ondines, mermaids, etc.

I saw two elemental queens of the water within the waves of the "Macuriba" (Atlantic Ocean). One of them had the color of coral and her tunic and face were of the same color. The other had a violet coloring. These beings looked like two splendid maidens and spoke in the esoteric language; therefore, it is necessary to practice in order to understand these beings. Really, they are of an extraordinary beauty.

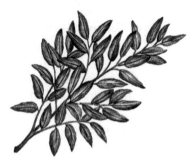

Eucalyptus globulus

The elemental kings of the water always use the trident (read *The Elementals* by Franz Hartmann).

The aquatic plants are the physical organisms of these beings. The lunar elementals possess a profound Neptunian wisdom. They build their homes within the bottom of the waters with ethereal matter. They intensely love, and they form many homes.

Mercurian Plants

The Mercurian elementals possess middling plants with yellow flowers, a penetrating smell, and varied flavors. These Mercurian elementals are utilized for mental magic.

If the human being wants to know about plants, then, indispensably, he needs to study our elementotherapy. Whosoever does not know about elemental magic can never know the power of the plants. Therefore, the botanists are nothing more than simple "charlatans."

The elementals are called peris, devas, dwarves, trolls, kobols, brownies, nixes, trasgos, goblins, pinkies, branshees, fairies, mossy people, white dames, phantoms, etc.

The elementals have body, soul, and an immortal, divine Spirit, just as the human beings have. In this book I only occupy myself with the superior elementals, even though there are millions of elementals from the inferior kingdoms. We leave those ones for the degenerated pseudo-spiritualists.

The ether, the fire, the air, the water, and the earth are densely populated by the elementals. There is a great elemental god at the head of each elemental kingdom, who governs and directs his legions.

The five gods who preside over the elementals are:

> **Indra**, Lord of Akash, or ether.
>
> **Agni**, Lord of Fire.
>
> **Pavana**, or Vayu, Lord of the Air.
>
> **Varuna**, Lord of the Water.
>
> **Kitichi**, Lord of the Earth.

These gods are the chiefs of the different departments of Nature, who govern and manipulate universal life. In order to manage these beings, one needs to be a master from the White Lodge, and in order to become a master one needs to have walked the complete disciple's path. Whosoever acquires power over these elemental gods has the power to govern universal life.

Venusian Plants

The plants of the Venusian elementals are sweet and pleasant to the taste. They possess beautiful flowers, happy and abundant grains. Their perfumes are always soft and delectable, and are employed in Sexual Magic procedures.

Solar Plants

The solar plants are aromatic and of an acidulous flavor. The elementals of these plants possess great magical, curative powers.

These elementals are called "sylphs" and they are the elementals of the air. The sylphs say, *"Where real worth is hidden, there the Sun's rays shine."*

They impress upon the student the importance of gaining what is called the consciousness of knowledge—that is to say, intuition.

The sylphs possess a formidable memory. As a result, they are wise. They remember the rituals and religions of the stars, and the wisdom from the most ancient books.

If the student wants to remember the ancient wisdom, the sylphs can instruct and teach him. The authentic astrologers inevitably have to know the rituals of the stars in order to manipulate sidereal magic.

There are also certain black magicians or black astrologers who communicate with black magicians from other planets by means of certain procedures of black magic. Thus, with that extra help and in combination with the planetary force, they achieve their evil goals. Those types of criminals are sure candidates for the abyss.

If the Gnostic student wants to practice sidereal white magic, then he has to purify himself and to study the rituals of the stars. These rituals are known by memory by the sylphs.

Whosoever does not know the rituals of the stars cannot practice the white magic of the stars, because the ritual is the instrument used in order to manipulate the forces. If the Gnostic wants to study those sidereal rituals, then he has to learn them from the higher sylphs (read the *Zodiacal Course* by the same author).

The sylph's appearance is like an innocent child. The sylphs feel horror towards the present "human beings," since they know very well that their "human" souls are "demon souls."

Millions of "human beings" already carry the mark of the beast on their foreheads and on their hands. Thus, the "demon souls" carry horns upon the forehead of their astral bodies, and on their hands they have a triangle with a point in its center. This triangle is the mark of the beast on the hands.

The authentic astrologer does not need to create amusement park horoscopes, as the style of certain astrologers who are already famous for their ignorance. The true master astrologer receives his teachings and indications from the stellar genii.

There is a temple in the center of every star. This is the abode of the genie from that planet. In order to enter into that temple, the true astrologer has to be a master, or at least a sincere and loyal disciple of the White Fraternity.

Whosoever can converse with the stellar genii does not need to make horoscopes, because the stellar angels show destiny to him. However, only the masters from the White Fraternity can be disciples of the stellar angels (read *The Revolution of Beelzebub* by the same author).

Nonetheless, those clairvoyants who are capable of understanding the esoteric symbolism of the stars are the ones who march on a true path of light.

When fixedly observing a star, the clairvoyant sees that the star is opening itself up into an arc. Then, the seer submerges himself within the aura of that star in order to "live out" all the events that await

him in anticipation. This is what is called authentic astrology.

The Plants from Mars and the Elementals of Fire

The plants that are influenced by Mars are sour, bitter, acrid, and fiery. Many of them are thorny and others produce irritation when touching them. Commonly, their flowers are red and small. They are found as small bushes that have a fervent smell.

The elementals who are influenced by Mars are the salamanders.

When we enter within the dominions of fire, we then enter within the dominions of the gods.

In Greece, the great igneous elemental known by the name of "Apollo" illuminated Greece's spiritual welfare and that of the surrounding nations through his oracles, which were pronounced by his Pythoness at Delphi.

The elemental gods of fire were the ones who inspired Joan of Arc. Sometimes they can impress many sensitive people to lead their nations out of moments of peril.

The great initiates speak with great reverence of those whom they call "Stillborn Children of the Flame." The redemption of mankind resides exclusively in the sacred fire of the Holy Spirit.

The Green-faced Man (who instructs one in the wisdom of the moon), the Beautiful Greek, and the Great Atlantean are some great gods from the fire.

We are going to transcribe a paragraph from the book *The Dayspring of Youth* by "M."

> History records many stories about the appearance of these elemental masters to the great men of the past. Here we

include a message from a fire elemental to a student:

"Before you were born I was acquainted with you in the inner spheres and we agreed to meet when you would return and harmonize yourself to my intelligence. After this long period I have come over to you in order to instruct you in the work that had interested both of us. The fire that you perceived today with your sixth sense was the signal we will always give you when we are here; for I have a following that will help and support you. We once spoke about your work at a time when you were born in Egypt; and I witnessed your insurrection in a certain province. You gained great power in your efforts to undermine the authority of the ruler under whose scepter you had command. You failed in this conspiracy and was decapitated. But you were able to win the interest of the great elementals of the fire mists. Much of your knowledge was locked; but we can unlock this and serve you faithfully."

- *The Dayspring of Youth* by M

The spiritual sun is pure fire and that sacred fire gives us illumination. The salamanders are small and thin creatures and their physical bodies are the hot plants that are influenced by Mars.

Whosoever learns to manipulate the elementals of the fire can cure many sicknesses, because everything comes from fire. The fire is the base of everything.

"**INRI,**" Ignis Natura Renovatur Integra (the fire renews nature incessantly).

Jupiterian Plants

The plants that belong to the Jupiterean elementals are of a sweet, soft, and subtle flavor, even though many times they hide their flowers. The Jupiterean trees are big and leafy, the flowers from these trees and plants are blue and white, with hardly any smell.

Saturnine Plants

The plants belonging to Saturn are always bulky and melancholic. They have gray and black flowers with a displeasing smell, and with acidic and poisonous fruit.

Also, the plants belonging to the Saturnine elementals can be heavy, without flowers. They reproduce themselves without seeds; they are rough and blackish.

Their smell is penetrating and their shape is melancholic and sad. The pine and weeping willow are Saturnine trees.

The elementals of the Saturnine plants are the gnomes or pygmies who build their houses under the ground and amongst rocks. They eat, sleep, live, and reproduce themselves as "human beings" do. Their bodies are ethereal and their appearance is like amiable dwarves.

Zodiacal Perfumes

Sick people must smell their zodiacal perfume on a daily basis:

Aries: perfume of myrrh

Taurus: perfume like costus root, an aromatic herb

Gemini: perfume of mastic

Cancer: perfume of camphor

Leo: perfume of frankincense

Virgo: perfume of white sandalwood

Libra: perfume of galbanum

Scorpio: perfume of coral

Sagittarius: perfume of aloe

Capricorn: perfume of pine extract

Aquarius: perfume of spikenard

Pisces: perfume of thyme

The whole organism of the sick person vigorously reacts when under the activity of the scent of his own zodiacal perfume.

Astrologers, magicians, and perfumers were always in the courts of Europe. Louis XV always demanded that his room be perfumed daily with a distinct essence. Catalina of Medici, wife of Henri II from France, relied on certain poisonous essences (which she slyly hid within her glove) in order to reject a suitor whom she did not accept.

Great healings with perfumes were performed in Mexico, India, Greece, and Rome. There are many books in the libraries of Spain that the Moors left behind in that nation. Those books contain innumerable recipes for odoriferous essences.

When Popea Sabina, Nero's wife, died in the year 65 A.D., Nero exhausted the whole Arabian perfume production for his wife's funeral.

The priests of "Tlaloc," in the country of the Aztecs, used the colors of the solar cult and a copal sack. The incense from this sacred tree was mixed with the vapors discharged from the hearts of their children, who were burned alive. This was done as a sacrifice to the Sun god. These Aztec magicians eagerly breathed in the spiritual forces from their incinerated creatures, with the purpose of incarnating within themselves those spiritual forces. These priests felt as if they were in the presence of the gods when they allowed this vapor to mysteriously act upon them... Nevertheless, this type of cruel and savage rite engendered a horrible karma for Mexico. Therefore, the arrival of the Conquistador Hernán Cortés to Mexico and the downfall of the Aztec civilization was the punishment that this people received because of such horrible and monstrous crimes.

There were many secret formulae of alchemy in the temples of mysteries.

The great masters from the temples in the Jinn state possess secret formulae in order to prepare perfumes. When their disciples inhale them, they then momentarily abandon their physical shape, or they are placed in the state of ecstasy.

These alchemical recipes have never been published because humanity would use them for evil purposes.

Elemental Magic

Elemental Evolution

Akash and Prana are eternal.

The incoming tides of "Monads" are dressed with vehicles when Prana enters into activity. Thus, they express themselves as "elementals." These elemental tides devolve and evolve. They descend from heaven, from Urania, and then they ascend again towards the infinite. This flux and re-flux of life eternally resounds with the Chinese "**kung**." Nature has seven elements that are populated by elementals.

The elementals descend from the worlds of light, downwards, until the mineral kingdom, and they ascend from this mineral kingdom, upwards, towards the worlds of light.

There are elementals from the mineral, vegetable and animal kingdoms. The most evolved elementals from the mineral kingdom enter into the vegetable kingdom and the most evolved elementals from the vegetable kingdom enter into the animal kingdom. The evolved elementals from the animal kingdom enter into the human kingdom. The elementals are eternal. A divine spark, the Innermost (Spirit), exists within every elemental. All of us human beings were elementals.

I, Samael Aun Weor, Archbishop of the Holy Gnostic Church, Master of Major Mysteries from the White Lodge, initiator of the new era and great Avatar of Aquarius, pronounce the following affirmations:

First, everything that Franz Hartmann wrote about the elementals is filled with very grave errors.

Second, everything that Leadbeater wrote about elemental evolution is filled with very grave errors.

Third, everything that the spiritualist writers have written about the elementals is filled with very grave errors.

Fourth, none of the evolving elemental surges could enter into the devic or angelic kingdom without having previously passed through the gigantic human evolution.

Fifth, no human being has existed who has not been an elemental. As well, no elemental current exists that will not enter into the human state.

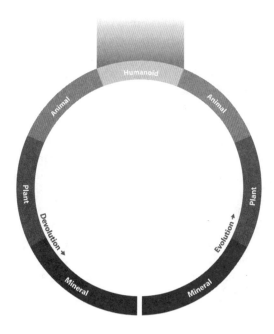

Sixth, if we clairvoyantly observe the interior of a rock, we will see millions of mineral elementals evolving within that rock. Therefore, the rock is only the physical body of those mineral elementals, just as plants are the physical bodies of the vegetable elementals.

Seventh, if we observe an animal we see that the body of that animal is the physical body of an animal elemental, who is preparing itself in order to enter into the human state.

We enunciate these fundamental declarations in order for the spiritualist students to open their eyes and abandon those horrible Theosophical and Rosicrucian Lodges that only produce degeneration upon thousands of souls.

There are certain elemental creatures with an animal appearance. One only needs to exert power upon them in order to unleash a tempest or to stop one.

The mineral elementals appear in certain places where gold is buried. They appear like a golden hen with her chicks, or as little golden children who soon submerge themselves into the place where the buried gold is located.

Every elemental has its own name. The name of every elemental is eternal. "Samitania" is a very ancient animal elemental whose virginal spark will completely awaken him in the future in order to incarnate him into a human body.

"Sereniyo" is the elemental chief of a group of wild pigeons that inhabit the hills of the eastern mountain range of Colombia. He has the appearance of an infantile figure with a suit of feathers and wings like a bird.

The elementals of gigantic trees look like giants.

The buried treasures remain guarded by the elemental guardians. These treasures are only found when the Lords of Karma command these elementals to surrender them. These elemental guardians can carry their treasures to other places and place them in a Jinn (enchanted) state. This is how no one can trespass the will of the Lords of Karma.

Egypt Elemental

The Egyptian civilization comes from a very remote Neptunian-Amentian period.

The Sphinx, which has resisted the course of the centuries, is simply the image of the Elemental Sphinx of the Goddess Nature. This Elemental Sphinx is the supreme master of the whole elemental magic of Nature.

When a master reaches the Fifth Initiation of Major Mysteries, seven paths appear before him, and he has to choose one amongst them (see pgs. 46-47). Devic evolution corresponds to one of them. The devas are the gods from the elemental paradises of Nature.

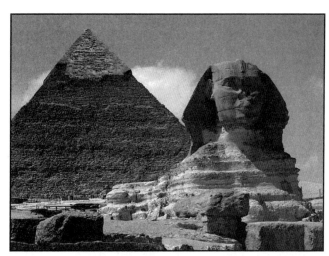

Agni, elemental god of fire, restores the igneous powers in our seven bodies throughout each one of the seven great Initiations of Major Mysteries.

The Goddess Nature herself is a "guru-deva" who governs creation.

Apollo, god of fire, guided the Greek civilization with his oracles, given through the mouth of his Pythoness from the oracle of Delphi.

Osiris and Horus were the great elemental gods from ancient Egypt.

We can study the great mysteries of the elemental magic of Nature in the college of the Sphinx.

The Guru-Devas work with all of Nature and with the human being. They are true masters of compassion.

Indra is the god of ether. **Agni** is the god of fire. **Pavana** is the god of air. **Varuna** is the god of water. **Kitichi** is the god of

earth. These guru-devas govern the elemental paradises of the Elemental Goddess of the world.

Medina Cifuentes, author of *Occult Treasures*, is mistaken when he absurdly affirms that the devas are not involved with human evolution anymore. The guru-devas work with the human being and with the elementals of this great Nature.

All the guru-devas look like truly innocent children. They live and play as children. They are disciples of the elemental Sphinx of Nature, who is the great master of these deva-children.

Masters and Disciples

There is a fundamental difference between those who have already reached the union with their Innermost—that is to say, the masters—and those who still have not achieved that union—in other words, the disciples.*

The master has the flaming sword. The disciple still does not have it.

The flaming sword gives the master a tremendous power over all the elementals of Nature. All the elemental populations of the earth, water, air, and fire tremble before that sword, which hurls fire and flames.

The master can simultaneously exert power over millions of vegetable elementals.

The disciple does not have that power, because he has not yet received the flaming sword. Therefore, the disciple must be meticulous and exact with the ritual of a plant, in order for the elemental of that plant to obey him.

The master does not even need to touch the plant. He can exert power over the elemental of that plant from remote distances, because the elemental of the plant trembles with terror before the flaming sword of the master.

It is enough for the master to unsheathe his sword at any given moment in order for millions of elementals to obey his command.

The disciple cannot exert such power over various elementals at the same time. He has to work separately upon each ele-

mental, by practicing the rite of elemental magic around each plant.

The master can command his Elemental Advocate to perform determined works of elemental magic. His Elemental Advocate will obey because he trembles with terror before the flaming sword of the master.

The disciple does not have the power to command his Elemental Advocate because he does not possess the sword yet.

---

* - The Human Soul (Tiphereth) incarnates the Innermost (Chesed) with the completion of the Fifth Initiation of Fire. The initiate can then be called a "Master." Yet, there are many degrees of Mastery. See *The Three Mountains*.

The Elemental Instructor of the Gnostic Medic

Every human being possesses an Elemental Instructor. This Elemental Instructor is made with the elemental substances of Nature and his creator was the human being himself. The human being created his Elemental Instructor when he too was an elemental.

The aspirations of the elemental-man engendered his Elemental Instructor. This is how his Elemental Instructor was created. The Elemental Instructor of the Gnostic medic is a master of elemento-therapy.

When the readers of this book want to exert a medicinal operation on a plant, they must request the presence of their Elemental Advocate and beg of it to practice the elemental rite of that plant, in order to join its vegetal element to the sick organ of the patient. Then, there is no doubt that the Elemental Advocate will join the vegetal elemental to the sick organ of the patient.

The vegetal elemental must be liberated only when the body of the patient is healed. Therefore, when the sick person is healed, beg the Elemental Advocate to execute the liberation of that vegetal elemental.

People who live in the city and who have to buy their herbs in the marketplace will practice the elemental rite around the cut plant, thus begging their Elemental Advocate to join the elemental of that plant to the sick organ or sick organs of the patient. The Elemental Advocate will join the fluidic cords of the elemental of that plant to the sick organ or sick organs of the patient.

It is astonishing to contemplate the vegetal elemental healing the sick person, rebuilding the sick organs of the patient.

Since the medicinal plants are millions, it is clear that our readers will need to be wells of wisdom, or Guru-Devas, to know all the elemental rites of all the plants of Nature by memory. Fortunately, each human being has his own Elemental Advocate of Nature, who has that elemental sapience.

Therefore, the Gnostic medic must train the person who will place the herb into the brewing pot to practice the elemental rite of that plant. This person will beg his Elemental Advocate to join the vegetal elemental to the sick organs of the patient.

This is the way our readers can join the astral cords of the vegetal elementals to the sick organs of the patient. Consequently, these sick people will be healed, because the plants are not the ones that cure, but their vegetal elementals.

Each vegetal has its own elemental. Therefore, there is the need to beg our Elemental Advocate to practice the rite of each plant. Our Elemental Advocate is the Elemental Instructor of Nature.

The Elemental Instructor possesses the supreme wisdom of the elemental magic of Nature. With his help we can open the storage and archives of Nature and learn the profound wisdom enclosed within the memories of the elemental world.

Whosoever receives the sword of justice has the power to direct his own Elemental

Advocate in order to make his Elemental Advocate visible before his disciples so that they can be protected against black magicians.

During Charlemagne's reign, many people and elemental beings profoundly entered into our physical atmosphere. It was precisely at that time when the romantic literature of the Round Table and King Arthur's Knights was born.

The great Elemental Kings of Nature live within a state of ineffable joy; they are creator gods.

Natural Magic or elementotherapy is as ancient as the world. The Lemurians transmitted this knowledge to the Atlanteans, who transferred it to the great hierophants of ancient Egypt.

If we consult history, we will become quite aware that the great men from the past studied under the protective wings of elemental Egypt. The great Greek legislator Solon, Moses, Apollonius of Tyana—all of them received their wisdom from elemental Egypt.

The foundations of the great Egyptian period are founded upon a very ancient Neptunian activity, which is based on the elemental laws of Nature. The Egyptians denominated this profound Neptunian consciousness with the name of "Amenti."

When the Gnostic medic affiliates himself with an internal school of elemental magic, he has to become skillful with the Astral Body in order to bring back all the memories into his physical brain.

There is a school of elemental magic in elemental Egypt. The student can affiliate himself with this school. This school is the temple of the Elemental Sphinx.

All of Nature is the body of a goddess who exists in the astral plane. This goddess has on her head a great queen's crown and

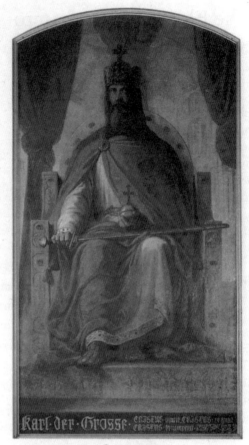

CHARLEMAGNE

she wears a resplendent white tunic. She is the one who commands in Nature; she is the blessed Mother Goddess of the world. She has a temple in the internal worlds, where she officiates and commands. This temple has two altars and in the midst of them we see a massive lion of gold, which symbolizes the "lion of the Law."

It is necessary for the magician to learn how to speak with this goddess in the astral plane. The Goddess Mother of the world also has her own Elemental Advocate, which is the Elemental Sphinx of Nature. The magician must learn how to command this Sphinx and how to converse with this goddess in order to become lord of all creation.

Hail Nut, eternal cosmic Seity.

Hail Nut, light of the Heavens.

Hail Nut, unique and primordial soul.

IAO, IAO, IAO, IAO.

Then the priest fell into a profound ecstasy and spoke to the queen of heaven, saying: Write thy teachings for us. Write thy ritual for us. Write thy light for us.

Then, the queen of heaven said in this manner: I do not write my teachings, I cannot. Nevertheless, my rituals will be written for all, yet only that part which is not secret. The law is like this, equal. One has to operate by the action of the staff and by the action of the sword. This should be learned and taught in this manner. - A fragment from the Gnostic Ritual of Second Degree

We learn the powerful elemental wisdom in the school of the Elemental Sphinx. This school is situated in the Astral world. Whosoever wants to be affiliated to it has to know how to travel in the Astral Body.

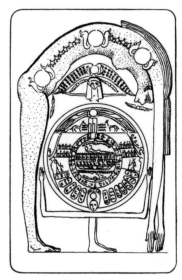

THE GODDESS NUT

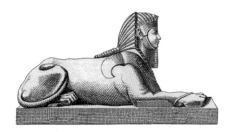

The Sphinx's image is just the material symbol of a great elemental genie of Nature, who is the single guardian of this very ancient wisdom of great Mother Nature.

When a Gnostic requests admittance into the Temple of the Sphinx, the Guardians meticulously examine him in order to see if he is worthy to deserve entrance and affiliation as a disciple into the school. Speaking in practical magical terms, this signifies that his spinal column is measured. For that purpose, the student is momentarily united with his Innermost (Spirit) and he receives the command to elongate himself in order to have his spinal column measured. Thus, if the guardian or tyler permits him, he will then enter as a disciple into the temple.

The Masons (from olden days) were disciples of this school of elemental magic. The master of this school is an ancient pharaoh initiate who teaches elemental magic to his disciples.

In this elemental Egypt, there is also the gallo or **GAIO** with his "**IAO**." He is an elemental god of Nature, who takes the shape of the gallo (rooster). If the disciple wishes to awaken his Kundalini, then he can beg this rlemental god of Nature and he will receive help, since this elemental master is a sage in the wisdom of the serpent.

This is why the gallo (rooster) could not have been missing from the Lord's Passion, since the gallo is the symbol of the sexual force. Therefore, the gallo of Christ's Passion is sacred.

The elemental atoms of Nature are Prana. All the elemental consciousness of Nature is Prana, or life. Therefore, whosoever speaks against the elementals speaks against life, and the princes of these elementals close the doors to him.

The elemental gods are impressive and mighty, especially Horus (pronounced "Aurus") who carries various bracelets or rings of massive gold around his forearm. When he delivers one of his bracelets to an initiate, then this initiate becomes a leader of a great populace.

The college of the elemental Sphinx of Nature resides within the very innermost parts of Nature. It is here where we are initiated and where the "codex" of the laws of Nature is presented to us. However, we must firstly pass a great ordeal, which in esotericism is called "The Ordeal of the Sanctuary." Very few have passed that great ordeal. Those who pass it receive a ring of a "monadic" substance on which the Seal of Solomon is engraved.

The Gnostic medic must learn to utilize his Elemental Instructor (Elemental Advocate) in order to cure ill people. The Gnostic medic must learn to manipulate the elemental substances of Nature in order to cure.

Prana is made with the most diverse elemental substances from Nature, which the Gnostic medic must learn to manipulate.

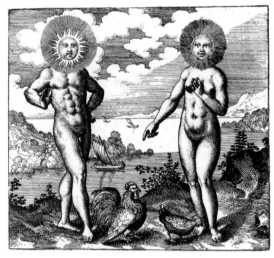

FROM ATALANTA FUGIENS, BY MICHAEL MAIER, 1618.

"The Sun needs the Moon as the Cock needs the Hen." An alchemical engraving demonstrating the ancient role of the rooster (gallo) as "he who awakes the dawn," the arrival of the Christ, the Sun, the Light of the World. The rooster is also a symbol of masculine sexuality, which can accomplish nothing without the feminine force (the hen).

Study and Exercise of Elemental Magic

Garlic Magic

Page 155 of the book *Occult Botany* (which is attributed to Paracelsus) has some mistaken data about garlic magic.

The Arhuaco Indians have known about the garlic's elemental magic since very ancient times.

The garlic shrub possesses various little, thin elementals with white tunics.

One has to bless the garlic shrubs before harvesting them. Five garlic heads must be harvested along with five leaves of "recrusada" and five leaves of the "carnestoledo" (*Cochlospermum hibiscoides Kunth*) trees. Each garlic head must be enveloped within a leaf of each one of these trees. Such leaves must be placed in a cross in order to envelope the garlic. Prayers of faith must be uttered while the garlic heads are enveloped. Then, all of it must be girdled within a little green bag. It is thus carried as an amulet or talisman around one's neck, in order to defend oneself

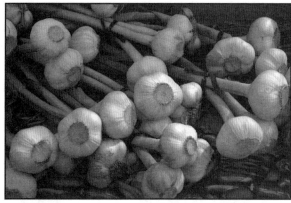

GARLIC

against the waves of evil, which are emitted by the black magicians.

Magic of the Artemisia Plant

This plant must be harvested at 12:00 midday on Good Friday.

First, the magician will trace a circle around the plant. He will then kneel before it. Next, he will pray, asking the elemental of the plant for the desired service. Afterward, he will yank it from its very roots and take it home.

The plant must be yanked while the magician is facing towards the east. By its roots, the plant must be hung on the ceiling of the house, so that the plant remains in a position with its roots aiming upwards and its branches aiming downwards. The plant must remain towards the east. The power of this elemental will grant unto its owner whatever was asked for.

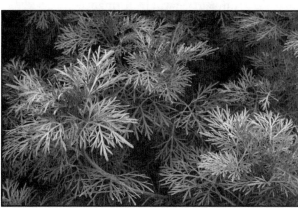

ARTEMISIA

Magic of the Angel's Trumpet

Datura Arborea L.; Known as Borrachero, Trompeta de Angel in Colombia and Mexico, Higaton in Bolivar, and Floripondio in Peru

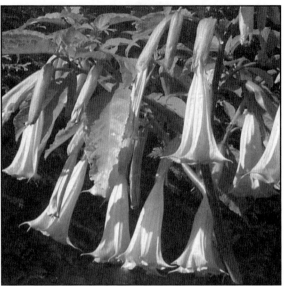

The elemental of the angel's trumpet tree is completely a magician. He is Neptunian and has tremendous powers. When clairvoyantly seen, this elemental looks like a twelve-year-old child. He carries in his hands the magician's magic wand.

Every angel's trumpet tree has its corresponding elemental, which has to be utilized by those who wish to consciously depart in their Astral Body. I was frequently utilizing the elemental of this tree in order to teach my disciples how to consciously depart in their Astral Bodies. I say that I was utilizing it because I am referring to ancient times.

Procedure

With a branch that I took from the same tree, I would trace a very wide circle on the ground around it. I would then crush the tree's flowers and dab the pressed juice from it over the head of the disciple.

Then, while lying on his bed the disciple would fall asleep; I then commanded the elemental to take that disciple out of his physical body. These commands were accompanied by the mantra of this tree, which is "**KAM**," and must be pronounced by prolonging the sound of the two last letters, like this:

Kaaaaaaaaammmmmmmmm

All of our Gnostic disciples of this day and age must employ the powers of this elemental in order to learn how to consciously depart in the Astral Body. For this purpose, simply proceed as we have just taught.

You must imperiously command the elemental like this: "When I call you, you will always assist me. I need you to take me out in my Astral Body every time that I command you to do so."

Afterwards, the disciple will pierce a finger of his hand with a needle and with a knife he will make an incision on the tree where he will deposit his blood. In this way, the pact with the genie of this angel's trumpet tree will be formalized.

> "Write with blood, thus, you will learn that the blood is spirit." - Nietzsche

> "Blood. Blood is a very special fluid." - Goethe

Then, the disciple will cut some hair from his head and will hang it on the tree. He will collect a few petals from the flowers of the tree and will place them within a little bag and hang it around his neck as a talisman. Hence, from that moment on, the disciple has under his service this humble elemental, who will always assist to his call.

When the disciple wants to consciously depart in his Astral Body, he goes to sleep on his bed and pronounces the mantra of this tree. His mind needs to be concentrating on this elemental genie, calling him mentally and begging him to take him out in his Astral Body. In the state of transition between vigil and dreaming, the elemental of the angel's trumpet tree will take him out of his physical body and will take him consciously to the places longed for.

Anytime the disciple can visit this tree he must do so in order to water it, bless it and to cut its flowers, which he will utilize whenever he wishes to do so. As we have already stated, these flowers must be crushed with a stone, then their juice is extracted and applied over the head in order to depart in the Astral Body. It is beneficial to warn that the application of this juice is performed at the time when the disciple will lay down to bed, when he is going to sleep.

However, when the flowers are not available, the disciple must invoke his serving elemental in order for the elemental to take him out in his Astral Body.

This elemental also has the power to make us invisible.

When the disciple wants to make himself invisible, he pronounces the mantra (**Kam**) of the elemental of this tree. He calls his servitor and begs the elemental to make him invisible. This will actually happen.

In ancient times, when I wanted to become invisible, I would crush the flowers as I already explained. Then, I would apply this pressed juice upon the joints of my body, while begging the elemental to make me invisible.

Nonetheless, we have to warn that what the disciple must first do is transcend his body. In ancient times, the human being lived within the bosom of Mother Nature. All of the powers of the blessed Goddess Mother of the world potently resounded within their resonant centers. Thus, these powers expressed themselves with the grandiose euphoria of the universe through all of the human being's chakras.

Yet, in this day and age the human being is completely unadaptable to Nature, and the potent waves of the universe cannot express themselves through him.

Therefore, our duty is to adjust our body to the bosom of the blessed Goddess Mother of the world again. Our duty is to clean this marvelous physical organism and to prepare our body in order to convert it into a resonant center for Nature.

Daily, the disciple must invoke the seven potencies with the powerful mantra "**Muerisiranca**" and beg them to prepare his body for the exercising of practical magic.

We must also be tenacious and persevering year after year in invoking the seven potencies, in order for them to prepare our physical body for the exercising of practical magic.

The body of a magician has a different vibratory tonality, different from the bodies of the other human specie.

No matter how good a musical instrument may be, if it is not properly tuned then the musician will not execute his melodies successfully. A similar situation occurs with the magician's human body. He has to tune his marvelous organism in order to execute his great works of practical magic with a plenitude of success.

The pressed juice of the flower from the angel's trumpet tree, when applied to the body's joints, is used in esoteric medicine in order to acquire agility in the muscles.

The seeds of this plant are only utilized by the evil ones for their criminal intents. We, the Gnostics, only utilize the pressed juice from its flower (petals).

We advise the disciples to have this marvelous angel's trumpet plant for their works of practical magic on the patio of their houses. Moreover, this plant is a guardian against evil entities.

Elemental Magic of the "Jayo" (Coca) Erythroxylum Coca Lam.

And was the word of Jehovah to me, saying, Jeremiah, what do you see? And I said, I see an almond rod.

Then Jehovah said to me. You have seen well; for I will watch over My word to perform it. - Jeremiah 1:11, 12

When we study these symbolic verses from the Prophet Jeremiah, we find that the almond rod represents the magician's rod.

In its purely vegetal aspect, the almond rod encloses a vegetal secret that Jeremiah did not want to unveil to the profane.

The "jayo" (coca) is hidden behind the almond rod.

This marvelous plant serves in order to help one depart in the Astral Body. The mantra of the "jayo" is:

Boya-boya-boya

There is a secret formula to prepare a potion with the "jayo." This potion permits the magician to consciously depart in his Astral Body. I must be very careful not to divulge this sacred formula, because humanity is not prepared to receive it.

Seyirino, father of the "jayo," is a great master from the Mayan Ray. The elemental of the "jayo" looks like a maiden of extraordinary beauty, with her body and her beautiful vestures made out of pure gold.

We, the Roman magicians from the ancient Rome of the Caesars, frequently used the "jayo" for our great works of practical magic.

Elemental Magic of the Juniper Tree Juniperis communis L.

The juniper is a very sacred broom tree. The Gnostic must learn how to manipulate the powers of this broom tree in order to converse with the angels. Let us now see the following biblical verses.

And Ahab told Jezebel all that Elijah had done, and withal how he had slain all the prophets with the sword.

Then Jezebel sent a messenger unto Elijah saying, So let the gods do to me, and more also, if I make not thy life as the life of one of them by tomorrow about this time.

And when he saw that, he arose, and went for his life, and came to Beersheba, which belongeth to Judah, and left his servant there.

But he himself went a day's journey into the wilderness, and came and sat down under a juniper tree: and he requested for himself that he might die; and said, It is enough; now, O Jehovah, take away my life; for I am not better than my fathers.

And as he lay and slept under a juniper tree, behold, then an angel touched him, and said unto him, Arise and eat.

And he looked, and, behold, there was a cake baked on the coals, and a cruse of water at his head. And he did eat and

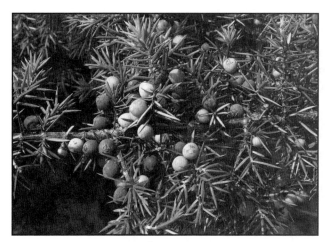

JUNIPER BERRIES

drink, and laid him down again. - 1 Kings 19:1-6

Biblical magic is something very holy. Very few are those who know it in depth. When the Bible tells us that Elijah sat under a certain juniper tree and that under this juniper tree an angel appeared to him, what is hidden behind this is very profound esoteric wisdom.

In order for an angel to make himself visible and tangible in the physical world, it is necessary to prepare for him a gaseous body, so it can serve him as a physical instrument. Therefore, the magician who wants to make the angels visible and tangible in the physical world must know the elemental magic of the juniper tree in depth.

The magician will collect some branches and berries from the juniper tree, which he will place within a container or pot with water to boil. He will drink a glass of that beverage when the ritual of angelic invocation begins. He will also place a censer over the altar of his sanctuary, in which he will put branches and berries of the juniper tree. He can also add branches of yarrow

(*Achillea millefolium L.*) for the decoction that he has to drink, as well as for the smoke offering in the temple. Yet, if he does not find the yarrow branches, the juniper tree alone will be enough for the rite.

The invoker must dress himself with his priestly robe. He can perform the ritual of First or Second Degree, or the Gnostic Mass as it appears in our book entitled *Secret Writings of a Guru.*

When finishing the ritual, the invoker will swing the censer three times, commanding the elemental of the juniper tree to form the gaseous body over the altar of the temple, in order for the invoked angel to make himself visible and tangible in the physical world. With a potent voice, the officiant must pronounce the name of the angel, whom he wishes to invoke, three times.

The Angel Israel can be invoked. The populace that now bears his name was ruled by him during all of the biblical exodus. Also, the Angel Raphael or the Angel Aroch, etc., can be invoked.

The juniper tree that was used for its branches for that rite must remain covered with black cloth during the whole ceremony. Some stones must also be hung from its branches.

The elemental of the juniper tree looks like a twelve year-old girl, and possesses great esoteric powers.

The branches and berries of the juniper tree also have the power of cleaning our Astral Body from any type of larvae.

This work can also be performed in a very simple way, within a room properly purified with frankincense and with prayer.

In this case, the ritual can be replaced with invocations performed with a pure heart.

The juniper tree will make a gaseous body that will serve as an instrument for the invoked angel. If our invocation is worthy, then the angel will come to our call and will make himself visible and tangible. Yet, if our invocation is not worthy of an answer, then the angel will not come to our call.

The altar can be simply made with a table.

When we read that the prophet Elijah sat under a juniper tree, this signifies that he invoked an angel by making use of a juniper tree. Thus, the angel answered his call and made himself visible and tangible.

The juniper tree has various mantras that must be pronounced during the rite. **"KEM LEM"** are the mantras of this vegetal elemental.

In the memories of Nature, we read that three zipas from Bacata practiced the rite of the juniper tree, in order to make the angels visible and tangible. All of the divine kings from antiquity practiced the elemental magic of the juniper tree in order to converse with the angels.

This marvelous elemental obeys an elemental queen of the fire. In the internal worlds, we see this great elemental queen seated upon her throne of fire.

The memories of Nature tell us that the juniper tree has the power of placing our endocrine glands into a special, super-functioning degree. This simply means that all the chakras of the Astral Body enter into activity by means of the rite of the juniper tree.

The elemental magic of the juniper tree belongs to the art of divine kings.

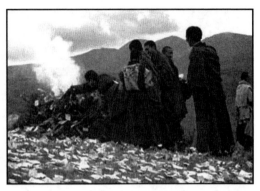

Tibetan monks write letters to their deities and subsequently burn the letters on a fire made of juniper branches.

We teach our disciples about great Nature's royal art in our book entitled *Igneous Rose*.

Igneous Rose is a book written for all those who are aspiring to enter onto the devic path.

In the book *Igneous Rose*, we deeply study the evolution of the elementals of the blessed Goddess Mother of the world.

In *Igneous Rose* we meticulously study the elemental magic of a thousand plants.

Therefore, all of those disciples who aspire to enter onto the devic path must study in depth our book entitled *Igneous Rose*.

We study in depth the elemental life of the earth, air, water, and fire in our book *Igneous Rose*.

There are seven paths of cosmic evolution, and *Igneous Rose* is the special book for all those who aspire to the devic path.

Maguey, Fique, or Cabuya
Agave americana L.

A great lord of the Light, a white magician in Lemurian epochs, wanted to stray onto the black path. I admonished him with advice in order to stop him, yet he insisted on going through with his intentions. Therefore, I was obliged to operate with the elemental of the maguey plant, who possesses great powers, in order for this magician to abandon that fatal decision.

I then ritualized in the already known way. Next, I cut one of the plant's fleshy leaves and I placed it between the palms of my hands, pronouncing various times the three mantras of this elemental from the maguey plant:

Libib, Lenoninas, Lenonon

Afterwards, I imperiously commanded the elemental to travel towards the dwelling of the white magician who was in danger of straying onto the black path. Thus, the elemental took the shape of a little goat and submerged himself within the magician's atmosphere, and accomplished the commands exactly as I had given to him, which was to disintegrate his evil thoughts and to fortify his good thoughts.

I also remember a curious case from the primeval times of South America. A father brought his son to me, who was a child of a young age. He did this in order for me to prescribe medicine for the child who had fallen grievously sick by pestilence. The child's fatal outcome was inevitable. Consequently, I told the child's father, "I will cure your child, but because he is already a lost case, you have to give him to me as an adoptive son."

The child's father agreed with my proposition. Thus, at that very moment I began to work with the maguey. I made the circle around it, blessed the plant and

pronounced its three mantras: ***Libib, Lenoninas, Lenonon***. Then, I commanded the elemental to cure the child of the horrible pestilence.

Afterwards, I removed the roots of that maguey and prepared a decoction. While the water was boiling, I blessed the decoction pot and commanded the elemental like this: "Work, heal the sick child." This is how the child rapidly recovered his health.

The elemental of the maguey plant is Jupiterian, and possesses great esoteric powers.

I had a reincarnation during the time of the government of the last Caesar from Rome. At that time I had fame as a magician. Hence, I was called by Caesar in order to help him get rid of a political personage, who was his mortal enemy. I accepted the job and operated with the elemental of the maguey plant. I approached the plant and blessed it. Then, I walked in a circle around it from right to left, cut one of its fleshy leaves and placed it between the palms of my hands. Afterwards, I pronounced the mantras of the maguey plant: ***Libib, Lenoninas, Lenonon***. I imperiously

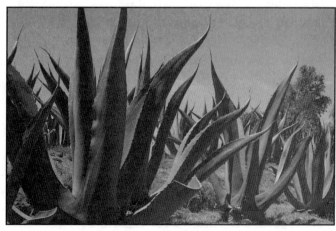

MAGUEY

commanded the elemental of this plant to transport himself to the abode of the Caesar's enemy in order to disintegrate his thoughts of hatred and to infuse into him love towards the sovereign. The results were astonishing, because in a few days the mortal enemies were reconciled.

Magic of the Guasimo Tree
Guazuma ulmifolia Lamarck.

The elemental of the "guasimo" plant is armed with powerful magical attributes. This elemental lives in the Tattva Tejas as a very distinguished elemental of fire. The cape that falls to his feet corroborates this.

The mantras of this igneous elemental are:

Moud, Muud, Hammaca

With these mantric words, the elemental of the "guasimo" is commanded to work for what is desired. The magician will take one of the branches of this tree, after having blessed it, and will trace a circle around it in accordance with what has already been taught.

Once the ritual has concluded, a bunch of its leaves must be collected and macerated for 15 to 20 days in a bottle of rum. Before starting the utilization of this medicament, do some passes with your right

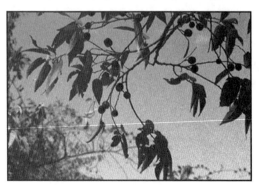

Guasimo

hand over the affected organs with the intention of collecting the diseased fluids, which must be placed within a sack made out of wool, because wool is an extremely efficient insulated material. The hand must be placed within the wool sack seven times for the already indicated reason. When this operation is finished, then close the sack's opening and pray to the elemental, so that he can cure the sick person. The Gnostic medic must perform this prayer while kneeling over a stone and when he finishes his petition, he will cast the sack from his hands with the fervent desire of throwing the rheumatism away from the body of the sick person.

Give the sick person a little cup of the maceration of rum every hour. The healing is quick.

Magic of the Gualanday Tree
Jacaranda caucana Pittier.

The elemental of the "gualanday" tree wears a dark green tunic. He belongs to the wisdom of the serpent.

I remember a very interesting case in those forgone times when the submerged continents of Lemuria and Atlantis were still united with South America.

A young female Indian who was the promised fiancé of a handsome man from the same tribe, was suffering horribly because of the consequences of a quarrel that threatened to frustrate the matrimonial agreement. Since I was the medic magician from that tribe, I was consulted by that grievous woman, whom I promised to help. Thus, I immediately operated with the elemental of the gualanday tree in the following way:

At sunrise, facing towards the east and with my head covered by a cloak, I approached the gualanday tree. Then, after performing the ritual that we previously described, I took two of its branches as a symbol of the bride and groom. Thus, with a branch in each hand and facing towards the place where the bridegroom dwelled, I pronounced the mantra of the gualanday tree three times:

Tisando, Tisando, Tisando

I commanded the elemental to transport himself to the residence of the bride and bridegroom to end the quarrel and to harmonize the couple. The elemental was not to abandon this assignment until such orders were accomplished.

After performing this procedure, I placed the branches of the gualanday tree over two wooden trunks that were on the ground. Then, I took the branches and whipped them against the trunks until the leaves became detached from them. I gave these to the bride so she could cook them with the groom's food. Thus, a short time after, the couple married and was happy.

There is nothing more efficient than the ritual of the gualanday tree in order to destroy the quarrels of marriage.

The elemental of this tree belongs to the wisdom of the snake. This elemental must be imperiously invoked and commanded in this manner: "**Tisando**, work intensely. **Tisando**, cure the sick person, heal his liver. **Tisando**, harmonize the marriage of (name), terminate their quarrels, etc."

The ritual must not be forgotten in the moment of harvesting this plant. It must be blessed and commanded to do whatever one wishes. Also, when the water from the decoction of this plant is boiling, the blessings and the vocalization of the mantra **Tisando** must be repeated.

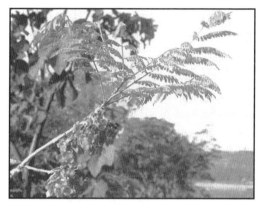

GUALANDAY

Dosage

In order to heal the liver, drink three glasses daily of the decoction of this plant before meals, for fifteen days.

Magic of the Guasguin Plant
MICROCHETE CONYMBOSA H. B. K.
To reconcile oneself with an enemy

This plant must be harvested during the day. A circle must be traced with a reed while over the top of the plant. Then, the letter "**S**" must be pronounced in the following way:

Sssssssssssssssssssssss

After having perfumed a cloth with the smoke of herbs, then the cloth must be blessed by making three passes in the form of a cross with "blessed water." Afterwards, it has to be perfumed with a fine rose essence, heliotrope essence and eau de cologne.

The assistants must keep themselves in chastity and must cleanse themselves from astral larvae. Therefore, they must practice Sexual Magic.

Magic of the Mammee Tree

Mammea americana L.; called Guanabana
Cabezona or Tutua Cabeza de Tigre
on the coast of Colombia

Collect nine leaves from this tree and make three crosses. Use three leaves for each cross; pin together the three leaves (with a pin) to form a cross.

One cross will be placed under the bed and the other two crosses as follows: one on the threshold (doorway) of the bedroom and the other outside of the bedroom's threshold. No black magician or sorcerer can enter into the bedroom when these three crosses from this plant are placed as indicated. This is the way in that many people can defend themselves from the forces of evil.

The magic circle must be traced around this tree before collecting the leaves from it. Also, the four cardinal points of the earth must be blessed while reciting the prayer of the Angel Gabriel, which is as follows:

Thirteen thousand rays has the Sun, thirteen thousand rays has the Moon, thirteen thousand times let all my enemies be repented.

The Angel Gabriel will reject all the visible and invisible evil entities with this prayer for whosoever performs this supplication at the foot of the mammee tree.

This tree has the thirteen powers from the Sun and from the Moon; therefore, it is very powerful. These thirteen powers are the following:

1. The holy house
2. The chorus of angels from Gemini
3. The thirteen candles that blaze in Galilee; the thirteen Marys

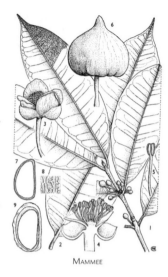

Mammee

4. The four tablets of Moses and the coffin
5. The five wounds (stigmata)
6. The six thousand chorus of angels (six holy barons)
7. The seven Pleiades that blaze in Galilee
8. The eight months and days of the pregnancy of Mary, who had the child in her womb
9. The nine commandments
10. The crown of thorns of Jesus Christ
11. The eleven thousand Virgins
12. The twelve apostles
13. The magical prayer

Those persons who want to reject their mortal enemies will trace a circle around the tree. They will then bless the four cardinal points and will recite the powerful prayer of the Angel Gabriel.

Elemental Magic of the Guava Tree 'Guayabo', Psidium guajaba L.

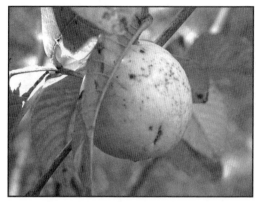

Guava

I remember something very interesting from those primeval epochs of South America, when Lemuria and Atlantis had not yet submerged. There was a lady who had been abandoned by her husband; she remained in a truly lamentable situation.

Feeling condolence for this poor woman, I performed a work of elemental magic with the guava tree.

I lit a big wax candle over a piece of cloth used by the husband. Then, I cut a branch from the guava tree and placed it next to the wax candle. Next, I imperiously commanded the elemental of the guava tree to bring into the house the absent husband.

This work was astonishing because the result was marvelous. The husband returned in repentance to his house.

The elemental of the guava tree resembles a girl wearing a pink tunic, who has a beautiful presence.

All of these works of elemental magic must be performed after having asked permission of the lords of Karma. Therefore, to all my disciples I teach how to depart in their Astral Bodies, in order for them to visit the temples of the lords of Karma.

When these types of works are performed against the will of the lords of destiny, then one falls into black magic and plunges into the abyss. Therefore, every work of practical magic must be supported with permission of the lords of the Law.

Those who do not know how to depart in their Astral Bodies can consult the lords of the Law by opening the Bible.

Before opening the Bible, beg to the lords of the Law, asking their permission in order to execute the magical work. Then,

with closed eyes, ask the lords of the Law to guide your hand. In an unplanned manner open the book, placing the index finger upon any verse of the opened page. Next, open your eyes and read what you have pointed to.

The Bible is highly symbolic; thus, the symbolic verse will be interpreted based on the law of similarities (analogies). The verse upon which we placed the index finger can be interpreted with a little bit of common sense.

This procedure with the Bible is done when we require direction regarding the execution of magical works, which act upon our neighbor's free will.

Elemental Magic of the Guarumo Tree Cecropia peltata

The "Mama" Kunchuvito Muya, an Indian master, told me that the "guarumo" tree serves as much for doing good as well as for doing evil, and also for healing sick people.

It is clear that we, the white magicians, utilize this tree for doing good. The children of darkness utilize it for doing evil.

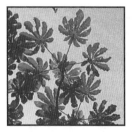 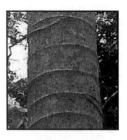

The "Mama" Kunchuvito Muya taught me how to cure sick people from far distances by means of the powerful elemental of the "guarumo" tree. He blessed the plant, then he commanded the elemental to cure a certain person. He placed a mug full of water close to the plant and put a stick within the water. Then, during the certain space of time he was stirring the water with the stick, his mind was intensely concentrated upon the sick person whom he wanted to cure from a far distance.

A circle must be traced on the ground around the plant in order to work with it.

A small vegetal host wafer enclosed within a cannula exists inside the trunk of the guarumo tree, as well as in its center. This vegetal host wafer can be used as an amulet in order to defend oneself against occult and invisible enemies, and also in order to aid oneself against the people who hate us. Carry this vegetal host wafer inside a small green bag.

Magic of the Male Fern

DRYOPTERIS FILIX-MAS L.

In the book *Occult Botany*, which is attributed to Paracelsus, we find a very grave error on page 183 regarding the magic of the male fern. The formula written in that book is mistaken. We believe that those errors were never written by Paracelsus.

Such errors belong only to his interpreters, successors, and translators, because Paracelsus is completely a master of wisdom. We, who have dealt with him, know very well that he is not guilty of these errors. Such mistakes were made by his interpreters.

The exact formula for the male fern is as follows:

On the night of Saint John the Baptist, which is the end of the 23rd day of June, at midnight (vespers of Saint John, June 24th), three persons will magically operate with the male fern. Such three persons must walk towards the place where the male fern is planted. They must go perfectly bathed, dressed, and perfumed as if they were going to a wedding ceremony or to a very fancy party.

They will place next to the male fern a fine cloth spread out on the ground. That cloth must be magically prepared with the smoke of the leaves of laurel, verbena, and "anamu" (*Petiveria alliacea Plumier*).

After having perfumed that cloth with the smoke of those herbs, the cloth then has to be blessed by making three passes in the form of a cross with "blessed water." Afterwards, it has to be perfumed with a fine rose essence, heliotrope essence, and eau de cologne.

The assistants must keep themselves in chastity and must cleanse themselves from astral larvae. Therefore, they must practice Sexual Magic; in their lives they must never cohabit (they must not live together frivolously).

The cleanse is made by performing baths with the plant called "mano de dios" or "lengua de baco." Do not mistake this plant with "lengua de vaca" (*Rumex crispus L.*).

The magician will trace a circle on the ground around this plant when the ritual is being performed. That circle must be traced with a branch from the same plant.

This plant has astonishing magical powers in order to reject the magicians of darkness. There is no black magician who can resist the whips of this plant called "mano de dios." Evil entities can be expelled from the house with that plant.

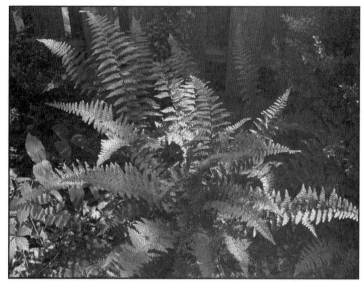

DRYOPTERIS FILIX-MAS L.

The magicians of darkness will terribly attack the performers of this ritual on the night of Saint John, in order to stop them from collecting the seeds of the male fern. Whosoever achieves the collecting of the seeds will fill himself with good luck and fortune. Money will smile upon him everywhere. This person will be filled with happiness and his business affairs will be triumphant. The whole world will envy him because of his fortune.

These seeds are only found on the day already indicated, at twelve midnight, under the roots of the male fern.

The assistants must distribute these seeds in a friendly manner, without arguments or ambition.

Every one must carry his seeds within a small jug, or better yet, inside a little bag and hung around the neck.

Extensive amounts have been written about this plant within the book *Tratie des Superstitions* written by the erudite Jean Baptiste Thiers. It is a book from the seventeenth century.

The powder of the male fern root is good in order to expel tapeworms. Consume ten grams of this powder within one hundred and twenty-five grams of water. After the space of one hour, drink a purgative.

Magic of the Jarilla Chivata Plant

The Saga Maria Pastora, who is a master from the wisdom of the Mayan Ray, taught me how to use the "jarilla chivata" plant.

The saga walked in a circle around the plant. Then, she blessed and harvested the plant. Afterwards, she crushed it and took the pressed juice from it. Next, within a container she mixed this juice with pure water and lemon. She gave this mixture to a young woman to drink who was sick with a pernicious fever. Subsequently, this young woman was totally cured.

The elemental of the "jarilla chivata" plant is a small and thin creature of a black color.

After the ill woman drank the potion and after the healing was performed, the saga sent the elemental away.

Magic of the Cashew Tree

Anacardium occidentale L.

The elemental of this tree has magical powers. If the magician wants a distant friend to appear or wants to terminate the quarrels of a marriage, then he must magically operate in the following way:

He will take the fruit of the cashew tree in his hands and say:

> **By the help of God, padoria, padoria, padoria.**

This mantra is pronounced with a loud, imperious voice, commanding the elemental of this tree to work over the mind of the person whom one is trying to influence. The skin of the fruit must be pierced with a pin during this magical operation. The phenomena will be mathematically performed.

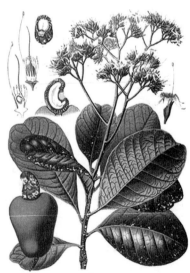

Cashew

I know in depth the psychology of certain 'super-transcended' people. When they read these lines they will qualify us as black magicians. Just as they do with us, they will do this with all of those who practice vegetal magic and elementotherapy.

If because we manipulate the elementals of the plants we are considered black magicians, then what classification should be given to the angels who manipulate the Tattvas by means of its elemental populations?

The manifested life is the expression of Monadic essences. These essences are compounded by focal essences, who are dressed with vehicles of distinct density. We call such focal essences elementals, human beings, gods, beasts, angels, archangels, etc.

Each plant is the physical expression of a Monad. We call these vegetal Monads "elementals." So then, who is the one who has the audacity to think that knowing how to manipulate the life of the vegetals is evil? How many ignoramuses who boast of hypocritical and cheap wisdom would wish at least to see (since they cannot exert power over them) the elementals from Nature?

Marvels of the Pine Tree

The pine is the tree of Aquarius and possesses great magical powers.

Cut off a branch that faces the rising sun and two branches that face the side of the sunset and form a cross with these. The body of the cross will be made with the one branch and the arms that form the cross will be made with the two branches.

Create an iron key during seven Holy Fridays. Leave a concavity or orifice in this key so that you can insert the stick of the cross through it. Whosoever carries this key will be exempt from any type of sickness that is produced by witchcraft. Also, any type of sorcery or work of black magic will have no effect over the one who bears this key.

The pine is the sacred tree of Aquarius. Every Gnostic must cultivate this tree in his garden.

Pine extract cures and purifies the lungs.

Pine cones (seeds) cure influenza. In order to prepare this remedy one proceeds in the following way: boil 15 to 20 pine cones in a liter of water. The sick person will drink three glasses daily of this ideal remedy.

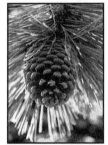

A Pine cone

Magic of the Roses

If there is human cruelty, it is true that there is also spiritual cruelty.

All of us who love the light have already passed through many types of "isms"; that is to say, we have known the schools of Theosophism, Rosicrucianism, Spiritualism, etc. Thus, where only love, brotherhood, fraternity and peace were proclaimed, we really only found hypocritical Pharisees, whitened sepulchers, resentment disguised within garbs of philosophy, terrible fanaticism and secret gossiping. Where we searched for wisdom we only found charlatanry, vanity, and stubborn pride.

There is no stab that hurts more than the one of spiritual cruelty. Thus, the poor souls who long for their superlative perfection and for their spiritual self-ennoblement suffer the unutterable on their journey, when they search for the truth inside all of those famous spiritualistic schools.

From those spiritualistic brothers all the infamies and scoundrely tricks are received. Yet, their worst cruelties are always disguised with philosophical phrases and sweet smiles. Hence, there is no stab that hurts more than the spiritual stab.

Moral sicknesses can only be cured with the magic of the roses. Therefore, all those people who are sick because of a spiritual stab can be cured with the magic of the roses.

Those poor souls who have a very deep emotional pain, let them be cured with the magic of the roses.

The rose is the queen of the flowers. The rose is influenced by Venus, the star of love, the morning star. A great ineffable master lives in that star. The name of this master is "Llanos" (pronounced *Janos*).

The chela (disciple) who wants to visit the morning star with his Astral Body will operate in the following way:

With his body well relaxed, he will lay down. He will get a little bit drowsy and then vocalize with his mind the following prayer:

> *Llanos... Llanos... Llanos...*
>
> *Help me, Lla... ma... dor... Lla... ma... dor...*
>
> *Lla... nos... Lla... nos... Lla... nos...*

Then, when the disciple finds himself drowsy (half asleep), he must sit up softly in his bed, throw the blankets off of him and get out of bed. Thus, once he is standing on the floor, he must jump with the intention of floating within the air. If he floats, then he must leave his house while floating in the atmosphere, pronouncing the invocation of the Master Llanos in the same way as when he was in bed.

The Master Llanos is an inhabitant of the planet Venus. He will hear the call from

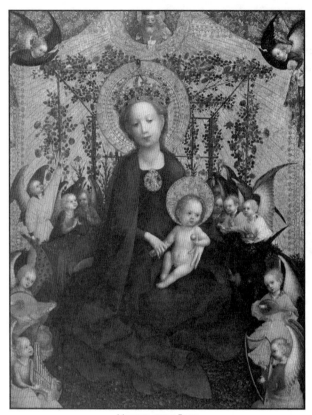

MADONNA OF THE ROSES

A guru once told me the following: "My son, this is a very dangerous hour for astral projection, because all the world is filled with a pink light..."

This master was right. If it is true that in the hour of Venus the positive ray from this star is filling everything with light, music, and love, it is also true and very real that the negative ray from Lucifer-Venus—that is the ray of the black magician Lucifer and of all of the Lucifers and tenebrous initiates from the copper cauldron—is also active. Yet, if the disciple lives a pure and chaste life, then he will have nothing to fear of the magicians from darkness.

Fortunately, Lucifer and the Lucifers have already fallen into the abyss...

This clue that we give here in order to travel in the Astral Body to the star Venus, I, Samael Aun Weor, received from the great Egyptian initiate Mary, mother of Jesus of Nazareth.

Tradition tells us that when Mary was making carpets for the temple of Jerusalem, those carpets transformed themselves into roses.

The lines from the hands of Mary, mother of Jesus, clearly tell us that she had a rich suitor in her first youth, whom she did not want to accept because her only yearning was to become a priestess of the light.

Mary suffered very much with the event of the Divine Rabbi from Galilee. She had only one spouse, who was Joseph the initiate, and only one son, who was the Divine Master.

the invoker (the llamador). He will help him in order to arrive to Venus, the star of the roses, the morning star.

The disciple will be welcomed by the Master Llanos when arriving to Venus, and if he wants wisdom, then the master will illuminate him.

The disciple will be overwhelmed because of the ineffable resplendence that springs out from the aura and from the diamond tunic of the Master Llanos.

This master has already united himself with his Glorian. Therefore, he wears a diamond tunic.

During the hour of Venus, the astral atmosphere is filled with a pink light of ineffable beauty.

Therefore, Mary was an authentic, pure, and holy Gnostic priestess. Her face was bronzed by the desert sun; her body was fine and agile. She was short in stature, slightly flat-nosed, and her upper lip protruded just a little. This master was humbly dressed. She had comfort in the first years of her life. Yet, later in her life, she was very poor. She used to wear a brown colored tunic that was faded and patched, since she was living in poverty.

Her holy life accomplished the most grandiose mission that can be granted unto a human being. Now, she, this prominent master, is reincarnated again in the valley of the Nile. On this occasion, she was born with a masculine body. This great soul came in order to accomplish a great worldly mission.

Magic Formula of the Rose to Heal an Emotional Pain

Place three crystal glasses filled with pure water upon a table, with one rose in each glass. These glasses must be arranged so that they will form a triangle: one glass towards the north, another towards the east, and another towards the west.

Each glass must be blessed by the person performing this rite, who will drink the three glasses of rose water daily in the following sequence: before breakfast, drink the glass of water that faces the east. Before lunch, drink the glass of water that faces the north. Before dinner, drink the glass of water that faces the west.

This treatment must be accompanied by a sincere supplication to the Innermost (Spirit) and to the White Fraternity, so they may help the person become free from the emotional pain in which he is situated.

Any emotional pain, as grave as it might be, will be cured with this formula, which is repeated for several days.

When and during what epoch has any physician cured sufferings of an emotional nature?

How many people die daily or get sick because of emotional sufferings? Nonetheless, it is sad to say that there has never been a compassionate person who has delivered to humanity the exact formula in order to cure emotional pains.

Cases of suicide are innumerable, and nobody has ever spoken about the magic of the roses.

Many certified physicians can be blamed for deaths that occur daily. Yet, human justice cannot reach them, even when, so to speak, they can fill up a cemetery on their own.

I knew young people who were humble and modest while they were simple students from the faculty of medicine. Yet, as soon as they received their physician's

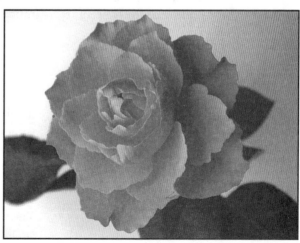

title, they became proud, vain, and despotic. Medicine is a very sacred priesthood. Therefore, by no means can a despotic or proud individual ever be an authentic physician.

The Queen of the Flowers

The rose is the queen of the flowers. When we investigate in the internal worlds the vegetal magic of the roses, we can evidence that the rituals of the queen of the flowers are our own Gnostic rituals.

There are some authentic Rosicrucian temples in the internal worlds. One of them is the temple of Monserrat, Cataluña (Spain) and another is the Temple of Chapultepec in Mexico.

The true sanctuaries from the true Rose-Cross order are totally Gnostic.

The Gnostic-Rosicrucian ray has its temples of mysteries only in the internal worlds.

The rose, with its immaculate beauty, encloses the most ineffable spiritual wisdom from the universe. The rituals of First, Second, and Third Degree are the Gnostic magic of the queen of the flowers. All the plants have their sacred rites. Yet, the sacred rites of the queen of the flowers are our holy rituals.

The Roses from Sirius

On one certain occasion, when I, Samael Aun Weor, was on the star Sirius, I saw from far away some trees that were each penetrated by a damsel of an ineffable and touching beauty.

Those damsels called me so that I could approach them. They were elemental damsels (nymphs) who were incarnated within

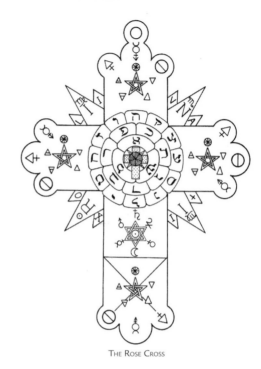

THE ROSE CROSS

those shrubs. Their melodious voices were music from paradise. I conversed with them, and then I withdrew, astonished with their plentiful beauty.

That planet has vast seas, and the inhabitants from that star have never killed, not even a little bird.

Their social organization would be magnificent for our terrestrial globe. All the economic problems from this world would end, and happiness would reign upon the surface of the earth.

The Sirians are short in stature, and they have all their internal senses perfectly developed. They dress simply with humble tunics and use metallic sandals.

Every Sirian lives in a small wooden house. There is no house that does not have a small orchard where the owner of the house cultivates his vegetal aliments. The owner of the house also possesses a small garden where he cultivates his flowers. Capitalists do not live there, cities do not exist there either, nor landholders. Therefore, the people from Sirius do not know hunger or disgrace.

There are some rose bushes in the garden of the great temple of the God Sirius that are unknown on our Earth. Each rose from that garden has various meters of height, and each one exudes a perfume that is impossible to forget.

The magic of the roses is something divine and ineffable.

Magic of the Sassafras

Sassafras officinale, Laurus sassafras

I remember a very interesting event in relation with the sassafras that happened in those far off primeval epochs of South America.

A certain indigenous person from the same tribe that I belonged to became filled with jealousy for his wife, whom he loved. He even reached the point of thinking that I, Samael Aun Weor, was making off with his wife. I clearly remember that while traversing a road, I encountered the

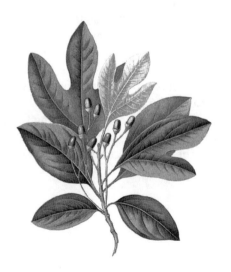

husband of this woman. When he saw me, he was filled with a horrible jealousy and he intended to attack me aggressively. However, he restrained himself. The man resolved to put the case in the hands of the Indian chief of the tribe.

I was the medic-magician from that tribe. Therefore, I knew in depth the magic of the vegetals, and due to that "scandal," I decided to defend myself with the elemental of the sassafras. The following day, very early, before the sun illuminated the horizon, I directed myself to the forest together with the woman who was the cause of that scandal. Some Indians were also accompanying us.

Then, when I located the plant called sassafras, I blessed it, I begged the elemental for the desired service and very slowly I yanked the plant from its very roots. This plant serves in order to end scandals.

Afterwards, I crushed the plant and extracted the pressed juice from it and gave this juice to the woman to drink who was the cause of the scandal. I also drank from this plant's juice, while my comrades silently observed us...

Subsequently, I stuck a spike on the trunk of the sassafras plant, I kneeled before it, and intensely concentrated my mind on the spike, commanding the elemental of the sassafras to transport himself towards the Indian chief and to dominate him with his powers. At the same time, while performing this magic work I was pronouncing the mantra or magic word of the sassafras:

Parilla-parilla-parilla

Then, the elemental of the sassafras plant transported himself towards the Indian chief and went around him while pronouncing his elemental magic enchantments. The elemental entered into the cerebrospinal nervous system of the Indian chief and totally dominated him by saturating him with atoms of love, light, and harmony.

So, the next day when I presented myself before the throne of the Indian chief, he was already in my favor. Therefore, I spoke with an arrogant and loud voice, "Why did you call me? You cannot act against me."

Then the Indian chief answered, "Enough with such scandals, withdraw yourself, you have no debts." Thus, this is how that painful incident passed.

The elemental of the sassafras uses a tunic of a resplendent yellow golden color. He is very intelligent, has a beautiful face, and his eyes are of a clear chestnut color.

The sassafras plant mixed with the juice of the plant called "sansevieria" (*Sansevieria zeilanica Willd.*) and "fioraventi" balm are used as a poultice in order to combat neuralgia.

The sassafras is also a diuretic and a cleanser. It must be harvested at dawn, the hour of the morning star, because this plant is Venusian.

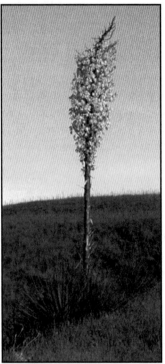
YUCCA

Magic of the Yucca Plant
YUCCA GLORIOSA L., YUCCA FILAMENTOSA L.

In magical terms, the trunk or center stalk from the yucca plant is called black hen (black yucca). The magician remains completely protected against the assaults from the Black Lodge when he makes a staff from the trunk or center stalk of this plant. Yet, this stalk must be cut on Good Friday at twelve midnight.

If this stalk with its leaves is hung from the ceiling, then the vampires (which are sent by the black magicians) remain stuck there.

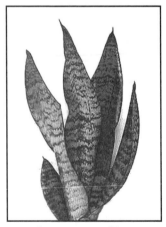
SANSEVIERIA ZEILANICA WILLD.

Esoteric Medication

The Secret of Health
Heal Yourself by Eating and Drinking

Having a plentiful life and sound health are two of the highest ideals of the individual and the species.

The most disturbing theme for all human beings is undoubtedly the theme of health. The problem of health disquiets everyone to some degree, whether they are wise or ignorant. Thus, during the continuous course of human existence, health has always been a problem for everyone.

Praised be the admirable plants that hide the virtue of health within their life and that offer it with generosity, as if they are fairies of love performing a gentle sacrifice.

Sudorific Procedures

1. While taking medicinal teas from sudorific plants such as sage, linden, and elder you must sweat in bed while well covered.
2. Take a steam bath for the chest and head by adding to boiling water four leaves of eucalyptus, four seeds of hemlock, or sage.
3. Place hot water bottles under the trunk of your body and legs and cover yourself up with blankets.
4. Take a steam bath for the chest and head while in bed.
5. Make a steam bath for the chest and head for small children.

Medicinal Tea

1. Cut the plants into small pieces.
2. Pour boiling water over the plant pieces. Let it settle for ten minutes.
3. Strain the medicinal tea through a strainer.

Decoction

1. Cut the hard parts of the plant and boil them on a low fire for two to five minutes.
2. Cover the medicinal tea and let it repose for ten minutes.
3. Pour it through a strainer into a tea pot.

Maceration

1. Cut any plant into small pieces.
2. Place the pieces into a glass or porcelain jar and add cold water.
3. Let it settle for six to twelve hours.

Dosage

3 to 5 years old, ¼ of a teaspoon.

5 to 12 years old, ½ of a teaspoon.

12 to 20 years old, ½ of a tablespoon.

Adult, 1 heaping tablespoon.

General Purpose Medications

Powerful Antibiotic of Universal Application

The parotidoicine is the most powerful antibiotic in the universe. Inject the microbe of typhus into the parotid glands of a fish. Then, reduce these glands to a powder and prepare it in ampoules or on slips of paper, according to what is wanted or needed for application. It has infinite application in relation with the sicknesses that humanity suffers.

Warning: The microbe of typhus is injected into the fish before it is dead. Then afterwards, the parotid glands are reduced to powder by means of fire (they must be burned). Then, this powder or charcoal is conveniently bottled, as we have previously explained.

Samael Aun Weor places medical science upon an absolutely new foundation with this antibiotic. There is no sickness—as resistant or unknown as it might be—that can resist the effects of this great antibiotic. This antibiotic was revealed to me by the Angel Aroch.

Bath of Beauty

Cook together barley, rice, bran, borage, and a sufficient quantity of violets and then bathe with this water in order to acquire beauty.

The ritual of elementotherapy must be performed with each of these plants according to the indications that we have given in this book.

Thus, the elementals of this formula will work in order to bestow beauty.

Danger of Contagion

Juniper berries are magnificent in order to avoid contagion. Thus, simply by chewing the juniper berries we can preserve ourselves from the danger of contagion.

Medicinal Elixir to Live a Totally Healthy, Long Life

A bottle of fine rum, one portion of juniper, two ounces of gentian, two ounces of rosemary, one ounce of cascara sagrada, two ounces of rhubarb, half an ounce of twenty-two percent alcohol:

Rhubarb can be acquired in powder or in tincture form.

Rosemary can be acquired as a vegetal branch.

Gentian can be acquired in tincture form.

Cascara sagrada can also be acquired in tincture form.

In case you are not able to acquire juniper, the elixir can be prepared without it.

I believe that this elixir can be consumed by little spoonfuls. Take three teaspoons daily.

Obviously, all the elements of this elixir must be mixed and then placed inside of a bottle.

I understand that the best rum is the one made from sugar cane.

Whosoever drinks this elixir must be very careful of not to fall into the horrifying danger of that frightful, abominable, repulsive, and filthy vice of alcoholism.

The Queen of Fire

The elemental queen of the juniper tree, who in the past times was reincarnated in an old medieval court, has tremendous magical powers.

The juniper plant is the vegetal from the solar dynasties. All of the divine kings from the past worked with the magic of the juniper tree.

The mantra or dharani of the juniper tree is "**Kem-Lem**."

The elemental of the juniper tree looks like a beautiful, innocent girl. Each juniper tree has its own elemental soul.

All of the elementals from the juniper trees obey this elemental queen, who in the past was reincarnated in the Medieval Ages, as we already stated.

The steaming decoction of the juniper tree (boiling within a pot) serves in order to invoke the angels.

It can also be used as a smoke offering. One needs to beseech Agni, so that he can help in the invocation.

During the rite, the invoker must drink one glass from this juniper decoction.

The chakras enter into activity with the rite of the juniper tree.

When burned, the berries from the juniper tree act as a smoke offering eliminating the larvae from the Astral Body.

One must ask the Father, who is in secret, to make the queen of the juniper tree attend to us, in order for her to help us in this magical work.

The invoked angel will materialize by means of the emanating steam of the juniper tree decoction coming out of the boiling pot.

When the angel becomes present, then ask the angel for whatever you need.

It is convenient for the reader to study my book entitled *Igneous Rose*.

The leaves of the juniper tree are marvelous. The tea made from the leaves of this tree helps women who are in their critical age.

The tea of the juniper tree is also good for the healing of the prostate.

The Virtues of Garlic

Garlic expels tormenting gas from the bowels.

When dissolved within wine, firewater, or tequila, garlic radically cures snakebites or vicious dog bites when it is applied as plaster over the bites.

Eating raw garlic or fried garlic softens the hoarse cough and clarifies the voice in an extraordinary way.

Purgatives

Castor oil is a magnificent purgative. There are also other purgatives for the cleansing of the stomach that do not cause harm. Examples: cascara sagrada, rhubarb, senna, etc.

Rattlesnake Medications

Deafness and earaches will disappear by applying to the ears the rattles of the rattlesnake, dissected and enveloped within cotton.

Uterine discharges are cured by receiving the vapor of a rattlesnake that has been placed upon charcoal embers inside of a vessel. The sick woman must keep herself away from any type of coldness and even from air currents. (EDITOR: see also Cancer.)

Tobacco

The pressed juice of the tobacco leaves (the leaves must be green), mixed with some fat and placed under the sun or over a gentle fire, can then be applied warm for colds, for the pubis, for pain in the side, on wounds and on tetanus, for whooping cough, on the abdomen, the spine, and sacro-lumbar area (for chronic diarrhea), and also on the navel of children for parasites.

To cure headaches that are caused because of cold, it is advisable to place tobacco leaves on the temples and forehead.

When hysteria and nervous attacks are present, the leaves of tobacco, humidified in firewater (liquor), are applied to the navel.

Tobacco is also used for epilepsy in the following way: one takes one ounce of good quality tobacco and cuts it into small pieces. It is then placed within a pot or container (with the quantity of one bottle of water) and is placed on the fire. After it is boiled for a while, one takes it from the fire and strains it very well and adds eight ounces of sugar. Subsequently, one places the pot on the fire again, until the decoction becomes like syrup. Consume two spoonfuls in the morning and another two in the night and drink half a glass of the decoction of the flowers of the elder tree after each dose. The sick person must stay in bed at least for three hours after each dose.

Also the CONJURATION OF THE SEVEN OF SOLOMON THE WISE must be recited with a lot of faith to the sick person.

On the front of the head rail of the bed of the epileptic person, place the magic

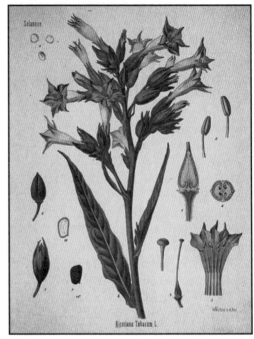

TOBACCO

symbol of the esoteric Pentagram, which makes the demons run away.

Epilepsy is a result of the Karma of the patient, who in his past lives served as a medium spiritist.

The epileptic person must never assist within nor ever visit any hall of spiritism.

Medications

Abortions

In opposition to the merely materialistic science and to the provoked abortions from this decadent and perverse era, the Gnostic medic not only pronounces himself against intentional abortion but moreover against accidental abortion.

Formula against Abortion

Twenty grams of powder of the root of bistort (*polygonym bistorta l.*), twenty grams of "grana de escarlata," plantain (*plantago major l.*), purslane (*portulaca oleracea l.*), coriander (*coriandrum sativum*), sugar.

There is no doubt that bistort and "grana de escarlata" are difficult to find in Latin America. Yet, the formula can be used regardless. Plantain, purslane, coriander, and sugar are not difficult to find.

None of these plants need to be measured. These vegetables must be pulverized and then mixed with a warm egg. The egg must be consumed; that is to say, it has to be drunk with these powders. This becomes a marvelous remedy against abortion.

The sick woman will remain in bed for forty days. The patient will take this remedy daily during the time of repose in bed. The ritual of elementotherapy, already taught in this book, must be performed with these plants.

Abscess, Dental

These abscesses easily burst by applying a poultice of leaves and shoots from the tomato plant, which must be alternated with another poultice of chamomile that is heated in a stock made from a hen.

For Aches and Neuralgia

Use "ferrobin" from the pharmacies.

Afflictions to the Sides of the Human Body

Make a decoction of honey (bee honey) mixed with goat milk. Leave it to cool and apply soaked cloths over the afflicted side. Afterwards, the sick person will take a purgative of almond oil. Upon going to bed, he must steam himself with the decoction of borage and "viravira" or, in its default, the decoction of contrayerba (*Dorstenia contrayerba L.*) will be utilized.

All of these simple and ancient remedies will be newly used by this modern humanity. When already tired and undeceived by chemotherapy and other sort of therapies, return into the bosom of Mother Nature.

Alcohol; Against the Vice of

This vice of alcohol can be cured easily.

FORMULA: Fry one or two owl eggs and give them to the drunkard to eat. The patient will be cured with this remedy. He will not drink for the rest of his life.

Another formula against the vice of alcohol is the turkey buzzard's heart. (Also called turkey vulture).

The turkey buzzard's heart must be pulverized. Put it under the sun to dry, before pulverizing it. These powders are deposited into the same drunkard's cup with alcohol, thus he will not drink alcohol for the rest of his life.

Amenorrhea, or Absence of Menstruation

Drink a water infusion of maidenhair fern (*adiantum capillus-veneris l.*) with wine, or receive vaginal vapors from the decoction of artemisia, or drink water from the decoction of chamomile. Also, beverages from the decoction of parsley roots, leaves, and seeds are greatly effective. Wine with rue (*ruta graveolens l.*), frankincense (*boswellia carterii*), and black pepper, administered in little cups, also produces excellent results.

Do not undervalue these remedies because of the modest way in which they are presented or because of their simplicity. The author has tested in various cases all of the formulae and works of practical magic contained in this book.

Remember that this is not a game for children, but a work for mature individuals. I, Samael Aun Weor, give testimony of my work.

Amenorrhea, or Suppression of Menstruation

Let a lump of sulphur be introduced into a bottle of rum. Afterwards, the following plants must be added: "contragavilana" (american goldenrod, *neurolaena lobata*

r.br.), "capitana," purple "guaco" (*mikania guaco humb. & bonpl.*), white "guaco" (*mikania micrantha hbk.*) and "malambo" (wild cinnamon, *canella winterana gaertn.*). The bottle must be then buried in a place that receives the rays of the sun during the whole day. After fifteen days the bottle must be taken out. The sick woman will drink it (in little cupfuls) until her menstruation appears.

Amoebas (Parasites)

In order to eliminate amoebas or parasites, macerate half a kilo of garlic and fifteen grams of Mexican tea or American wormseed (*chenopodium ambrosioides l.*). In South America, this plant is known by the name of "paico."

Bury the bottle (one big liter) in a place where the sun is always heating the soil. This bottle must remain buried for twenty days.

Before receiving this medicine, the patient must submit himself to fasting for three days.

During this fasting, the patient will eat sweets. On the third day, while fasting, he will consume one cup in the morning, and another cup at night. Do this for three consecutive days, thus the patient will eliminate the amoebas.

Anemia

Squeeze the juice from one beet and mix it with the same quantity of orange juice. The patient will consume this in the morning on an empty stomach, for nine days each month.

Anemia

Ferrous sulfate.

Anemia, Tropical

This horrible sickness is due to impoverishment of the blood. The blood is filled with white cells, and day after day the red cells are decreasing. This is the reason why anemic people present a yellow color in their flesh, extreme weakness, nervousness, cardiac palpitation, etc.

The first thing that these patients must do is to clean their stomach with a good laxative. Then, afterwards, they must be treated with a hepatic extract (injected and oral).

If the case is very grave, the anemic person must start with one hepatic extract ampoule of 1 c.c., and then increase the dose daily, until reaching 5 c.c. This treatment is for six months. Thus, the healing will be effective.

Note: The hepatic extract is prepared in the following way.

Put one pound of fresh liver into a double boiler and heat for approximately a two-hour period. Then, remove the pot from the stove in order to bottle up the hepatic extract.

Once the previous treatment is completed, the sick person must rehabilitate himself with the following restorative:

Wine for consecration	1 bottle
Citrate of iron	2 grams
Tincture of boldo	2 ounces
Tincture of gentian	2 ounces
Tincture of rhubarb	1 ounce
Tincture of quinine	1 ounce
Tincture of cinchona	1 ounce
Cream of tartar	1 ounce
Neutral glycerin	5 grams
Hepatic extract	3 ounces

The sick person will drink from this marvelous restorative, one small cupful each hour, being confident that the sickness is disappearing.

Angina Pectoris

Administer through injection four hundred thousand (400,000) units of penicillin every three hours. Take three grams of powdered sulfatiasol and three grams of powdered sulfadiazina, mixed with honey (bee honey). Gargle with it and also do "coluctorios" for the larynx.

Angina (Sore Throat)

1. Take a bath towel and fold it into four parts. Then submerge it into cold water and take it out without squeezing the water out of it.

2. Keep in mind that before performing the former operation, there is the need to soak the floor with an abundant amount of water. Your first step must be made with your right foot.

3. Thus, the towel folded into four parts is placed within the water and then picked up while water pours out from it, in order to execute a friction operation. First, rub the right leg (with the towel) from the hip down.

4. Take the other side of the towel and repeat the operation of placing it within the water and picking it up as water pours out of it, in order to execute the friction operation on the left side. Understand that the left side means from the

waist or hip towards the bottom of the leg.

5. Now, fold the towel in order to expose the unused sides and again repeat the operation of placing it within the water and picking it up while water pours out of it, in order to execute the friction operation from the right shoulder down, including half of the back and also the right arm.

6. Now, take the other side of the towel, the side that has not yet been used and repeat the operation of placing it within the water and picking it up as water pours out of it and perform the same friction on the left side, from the left shoulder down.

7. At this point, fold the towel in order to expose the other unused sides and repeat the operation of placing it within the water and picking it up while water pours out of it. Now apply it along the body, from the head down, counting from one to ten.

8. The patient must then put on a robe and apply mud all over the soles of his feet and throat.

9. Cover the legs and feet of the patient all the way up until ten centimeters above his knees.

The legs must be covered up with a wet or wrung out bed sheet. Half of the sheet must be wet and the other half dry. The half that is wet is used in order to cover up the legs. The other dry half will then be used in order to cover up the wet part, thus covering the legs with both the wet and the dry parts of the sheet.

Then, this complete envelopment will be covered up with a big dry bath towel. Thus, this is the way in which the patient will sleep for the entire night.

This leg covering, along with the mud, will be taken away in the morning and the patient will rest until his body recuperates its normal temperature.

10. Then, repeat the whole friction operation, but this time the towel must be wrung out (not drenched). Thus, the patient will be placed again in the bed for half an hour to an hour.

With this treatment the patient will be alleviated.

RECOMMENDATIONS

We advise the patient to always keep his legs more covered from his knees down and to sleep more covered from his waist down.

This treatment, which is complex in its explanation, becomes very simple in practice.

Aphthas (Canker Sores)

Children sometimes get small white spots or pustules in their mouth that are very hard to get rid of. Yet, they can be taken away with the following recipe. A sweet syrup must be prepared as follows: a square centimeter of borax or atincar syrup, 25 grams of borax, and two and a quarter pounds of sugar, diluted within one liter of water and put to boil.

Aphthas

The teas or beverages of walnut are marvelous in order to radically cure aphthas. Bless the walnut tree and beseech your Elemental Advocate (whom you carry inside, within your Innermost Being), to work with the elemental of the walnut tree so that this elemental can cure the aphthas.

Aphtha / Thrush

With strokes of a brush, apply the pulpy juice of blackberries with boric acid, only on the part where the aphtha/thrush is located. Repeat the application various times. This will be sufficient in order to cure the child.

Apoplexy, Asphyxia, Lethargic Fever, Spasmodic Colic, and Difficult Parturition

The decoction of tobacco is very efficient in those cases perfectly defined as apoplexy, asphyxia, lethargic fever, spasmodic colic, and difficult parturition.

In all these cases, boil the tobacco leaves and administer enemas of this decoction to the patient.

Appendicitis, Acute

Boil the "espaletaria" plant (search in plant stores), mountain arnica, a spoon of powdered "piona" seed (it is a red seed with black which is used for children; it is a liana plant).

Arteriosclerosis

Arteriosclerosis can be cured with vegetal teas of: garlic, "siete sangrias," guaiacum (*guaiacum officinale*), "espinillo," mistletoe, fumitory (*fumaria officinalis l.*), dog rose (*rosa canina*), etc.

These plants must be boiled and the patient must drink the tea as an ordinary beverage until the sickness disappears.

Any of these plants cure arteriosclerosis. If the sick person becomes tired of drinking the tea of one plant, then he can continue with another. Then, at the end, he chooses the plant that makes him feel better.

Asthma

This sickness is radically cured with the following formula:

Water	1 liter
Goat manure	a sufficient quantity
Borage (*borago officinalis*)	one little branch
Hard, burnt sugarcane (*panela*)	
	a sufficient quantity

Within a proper container, melt the hard sugar cane (panela) upon the fire. The borage and the goat manure are decocted in a separate container. The mixture of the whole remedy is bottled up within a bottle. Take a spoonful of it every hour until it is no longer necessary.

Even when the sickness of asthma has disappeared in its characteristics and acute manifestations, this does not signify that the sickness has completely extinguished itself. This is because a membranous bag remains adhered to the bronchi, which is necessary to throw away in order to avoid future attacks. This can be done by adding the plant known by the name of "sipaca" ("papunga"), to the already described treatment. This new combination with the "sipaca" plant will be performed only after the first treatment has produced its healing effects.

As in all cases described in this book, the harvesting of these plants will be performed after having blessed them and after having commanded the respective elemental to execute the healing.

It may cause repugnance and it may seem strange to the allergic, sick people that we use animal manure in some of our formulae. Nonetheless, the healing possibilities of many sicknesses that are called incurable could not be cured without the healing properties of animal manure (as is the case with goat manure); this excuses us its use in our various formulae. Pain and suffering do not have extreme social refinements, nor wrongly defined "cleanliness." If the suffering that suppresses us incites us to expect death with gladness, why not make the sacrifice in order to live sanely through natural, secure, and obvious ways?

Another very efficacious formula that can be used, in case the former one is lacking, is the following:

Antypirine	10 centigrams
Caffeine	half a gram
Acetate of quinine	half a gram
Tincture of aconite	quarter of an ounce
Tincture of nux vomica	
	quarter of an ounce
Tincture of boldo	half an ounce
Tincture of rhubarb	half an ounce
Sulfate of magnesia	3 ounces
Sulfate of soda	3 ounces
Water	350 grams

Take three small cupfuls daily, one before every meal.

Bear lard decocted along with sweet basil and mint or castile mint is also advisable for the asthmatic attacks. DOSAGE: A spoonful every hour.

In the acute period of this sickness, in order to shorten its attacks, an ampoule of 2 c.c. of adrenaline must be administered.

Asthma

(When asthma comes as a result of a sunken rib, surgery is then required).

> 30 grams of borage (*borago officinalis l.*) In branches (it can be acquired in herbal stores).
> 15 Grams of eucalyptus (leaves).
> 30 Black droppings (crushed) of goat manure
> 1 ½ Liters of water.

Place everything to boil for five minutes. Then, drain the decoction in order to take the sediments out.

Afterwards, in a pan or another similar utensil, bring to boil a quarter of a "panela" (hard sugar cane) until it is burned. Stir it, so it can be evenly burned. Then, when the smell of the burned hard sugar cane is present, add to it, little by little, small spoonfuls of the already drained water, with the purpose of softening the hard sugar and adding to it the already drained preparation. The result will be a type of tinted wine (if it dyes something, the mark will not come out).

Add to this preparation benzoate of soda (a quantity that can fit on the tip of a knife) with the purpose of avoiding the fermentation of this preparation and also for the good of the asthmatic person's illness.

This treatment must be performed for ninety days, even if the asthmatic person is cured in fifteen days, in order to avoid the return of the illness. This medicament acts as a laxative, therefore four spoonfuls or little cupfuls will be administrated everyday. The dosage must be decreased only when the digestive system has become too loose. The dosage for children is cut in half, according to their age.

Bottled beverages must be avoided, as well as ice cream, ice, and everything that can cause damage if one has a common cold.

Asthma

Asthma can be cured with the following plants: "ohaoteooc cocche" and "belinooc," the cooked hot bark of "petezcuch" (Mexican plants).

Grind these with five "escures." Drinking this in the morning, on an empty stomach, will cure the asthmatic person.

Asthma

Asthma is a horrible sickness that has killed many people.

This ominous sickness is cured with the pressed juice of the cabbage plant.

Add two egg yolks from a hen, shells and all, then sweeten the remedy with honey (bee honey), at least half a glass of honey.

It is necessary to boil all of these elements as best as possible and to take off the foam that rises to the top.

Then, add saffron and even a spoonful of fine sugar. There is the need to cook and prepare this syrup very well until it acquires a good consistency.

I believe that a little bit of sodium benzoate must be added to the syrups, no matter which syrup it is, so that they do not ferment. However, the quantity of that substance should only be an amount that can be taken with the tip of a knife. This is what signifies "a little bit" of sodium benzoate. However, sodium benzoate will not be necessary if the syrup can be kept properly stored within the refrigerator.

It is clear that the syrup will be very well preserved in this condition, without the necessity of adding sodium benzoate. Therefore, sodium benzoate is not necessary. Everything depends upon the way in which we can preserve this syrup.

Asthma

Drinking teas of the following medicinal plants can cure this distressing and terrible sickness:

"Quebracho blanco" (*astronium spp.*), "ambay," juniper, lavender, st. john's wort (*hypericum perforatum l.*), lobelia, pine, milkwort (*polygala senega l.*), horehound (*marrubium vulgare l.*), "chachacoma" (*escallonia tubar l.*), "chañar."

INDICATIONS:

All of these plants (which are used in distinct medicinal teas) do not have exact measurements, nor are they prescribed in grams. Therefore, any of these plants can be used for a tea; just cook them, that is all.

Whosoever studies this book scrupulously will know how to use the elementals. One must have faith in God, in the angels, in the elementals, and in all that is divine.

We have already taught that every plant is the physical body of an elemental of Nature.

It is clear that the Gnostic medic must always ask his Father, who is in secret.

The Father commands the Elemental Advocate, who commands the elemental of the plant, so that the plant elemental can cure the patient.

Faith performs prodigies and marvels.

Against Bad Breath

Seventy-five grams of coffee very well toasted and pulverized, twenty-five grams of charcoal reduced to powder, twenty-five grams of pulverized boric acid, twenty-five grams of saccharine, twenty-five grams of tincture of vanilla and enough quantity of gum mucilage.

The patient must consume six tablets daily. This is how the bad breath will totally disappear.

There is no doubt whatsoever about the damage that bad breath originates in the world of social relations. Even though it seems incredible, bad breath can be the reason for lost opportunities and business for the one who possesses it, due to the repugnance it causes our fellowmen.

If you suffer from bad breath, then eliminate it with the formula we give here for you.

Baldness; Danger of Becoming Bald

Against the danger of becoming bald, a very simple formula exists:

Half a liter of firewater or tequila, one small spoonful of salt, one gram of cinchona or peruvian bark. It is necessary to leave this in infusion for fifteen days before using it.

Rub the scalp of your head with this remedy every night before going to sleep.

This is how your hair will stop falling out before reaching total baldness.

Belly, to Decrease the

Drink a decoction of dutchman's pipe (*aristolochia tomentosa sims*), artichokes, and purslane (*portulaca oleracea l.*) regularly, as if drinking water.

Bladder

For illnesses of the bladder, the following teas can be drunk: "alfilerillo," spanish broom (*spartium junceum l.*), "calaguala" (*polypodium glaucophylum kze.*), "gramilla," boxwood (*buxus sempervirens l.*), salsify (*tragopogon porrifolius l.*), "doradilla" (*chaetolepis microphylla*), watercress (*nasturtium officinalis*), red currant or wild gooseberry, corn silk, dandelion, horsetail (*equisetum arvense l.*), etc.

Any of these plants make a good medicinal tea for the bladder.

Bladder

Cure the bladder by consuming three daily glassfuls of the decoction of horsetail (*equisetum arvense l.*). The first one must be taken in the morning on an empty stomach.

Bladder Pain

The pains in the bladder disappear with enemas of the following plants: common plantain (*plantago major l.*) and horsetail (*equisetum arvense l.*).

Within two liters of water put fifteen grams of either of these two plants. When this water is at the body's temperature, then perform two or three intestinal baths (enemas). The decoction of these two plants can also be consumed.

Blood; A Great Cleanser for the

For the space of fifteen days, bury in a very sunny place a bottle of rum into which some quantity of carob tree bark has been mixed. Then, at the end of the fifteenth day take the bottle out. Thus, the cleanser will be ready. This will be consumed by little cupfuls, one every hour.

Blows and Contusions to the Head

One ounce of sea salt, three ounces of very pure honey (bee honey), two ounces of turpentine, and three cumin seeds: If these are mixed with great patience over a low fire, then a magnificent medicine will be obtained against blows and contusions to the head.

One makes a poultice with this remedy, which must be applied hot to the painful area of the head.

Then, the blow will not swell up and it will become totally healed.

Swollen Breasts

Place a half bottle of white wine within a pot, a good quantity of honey (bee honey) and twelve egg yolks.

Cook this preparation very slowly, keeping the pot always very well covered.

The breasts will be totally healed with this remedy.

What is important is to have patience and constancy in the rubbing application of this medicine, until becoming healed.

Bronchial Catarrh

Red poppy (*papaver rhoeas l.*), green onion, eucalyptus, flaxseed, and mallow (*malva sylvestris l.*): consume the decoction of these plants four times a day.

Bruises

The tree called "ararat" serves in order to cure bruises, especially bruises on the knees.

Bruises; Against Contused Wounds

Take a bunch of arnica (*arnica montana l.*) and another of horsetail (*equisetum arvense l.*). Boil them very well in water until they become very well concentrated and then mix with clay. Next, apply this warm on the area affected by the bruise. This water can also be drunk three times a day.

Burns

The following formula serves to treat burns: crush the white part of a green onion (the big headed onion is not good for this), add earth soap or mountain soap (the natural soap that is made in rural regions), add a little bit of salt and make a plaster, then dab it over the burned area. Afterwards, pour cooking oil over the burned area; it is better if it is olive, almond, or fig oil.

Burns

With maximum hastened urgency it is necessary to take a little bit of raw mineral lime and place this within water for the space of two hours.

When the lime is resting on the bottom and the water becomes clear (although slightly dyed white), then filter it through a piece of cloth, filter, or strainer, so that only the dyed water will remain and not the lime.

This marvelous water must be mixed thoroughly with fresh pork lard.

Blend this as best as possible, in order to make a magnificent pomade.

You can keep this inside of a cup and any time you need to use it, you will skillfully extend a little bit of lard on a piece of gauze and apply it to the burn, finally tying it with a band. This healing application must be applied on the patient every three hours.

Thus, this is how the patient will be healed from the horrible burns. By no means should this type of healing be suspended, not until the patient is healed.

Calculi; Remedy to Eject Stones from the Kidneys and Bladder

A sufficient amount of the thin skin or shells from fava beans, a sufficient quantity of marshmallow (*althea officinalis*) and pellitory-of-the-wall (*parietaria diffusa* or *p. officinalis*): within a pot, cook all of this very well in water and give this water to the sick person to drink as an ordinary beverage.

It is convenient for the patient to first take a purgative before using this medicine. It is necessary to ritualize to the elementals of these plants before using them, such as we have taught in elementotherapy.

Calculi, Gall Bile

Cascara sagrada (*rhamnus purshiana dc.*)	
"Fidico" extract	one ounce
Rhubarb (*rheum spp.*)	one ounce
Boldo (*peumus boldo*)	one ounce
Red cinchona (*cinchona succiruba*)	one ounce
Gentian (*gentiana lutea*)	one ounce
Senna	one ounce
Artichoke	one ounce

(If the ounce of artichoke is not easily obtained, then buy an artichoke in the market, boil it and get one ounce)

Consume three small spoonfuls diluted within panela (hard sugar cane) water, tomato juice or grape juice, three times a day. This recipe ejects the gall bile calculi.

Calculi, Gall Bile, Another Recipe

One hundred seeds from the fruit of the medlar tree (*mespilus germanica*), the white part, one quarter of a liter of olive oil: Liquify this and drink it in little cupfuls on an empty stomach.

Calculi; Biliary or Gallbladder Stones

These are expelled by placing within a glass the measurement of three fingers worth of extra virgin olive oil and three fingers worth of lemon juice. Mix it and drink it when the stomach is empty, before going to sleep. In the morning, take the same dosage again on an empty stomach. Do not consume anything with salt; drink only juices the whole day.

Calculi of the Gallbladder

Against gallbladder stones, teas from the following plants are good: knotgrass (*polygonium aviculare l.*), boldo (*peumus boldo*), "gramilla," rhubarb, "espina colorada," horsetail (*equisetum arvense l.*), "cepa de caballo," arenaria rubra l., "combreto," etc.

These teas must be drunk with a lot of faith.

Calculi of the Gallbladder, Lack of Appetite, Sourness, and All Type of Aches Within the Digestive Tract

Behold here, beloved reader, one of the most marvelous plants. However, because of its abundance and simplicity, we have not recognized the importance it possesses. All of its medicinal powers place it on the summit of all plants and it can very well take part in the teamwork of sacred plants referred to by the great Master Guru Huiracocha.

That plant is the medlar (*mespilus germanica*). Following, we give the exact method of how this plant must be employed, because if it is not done in the indicated way, it will not give the desired results.

Take about ten seeds from very well ripened medlar fruits, with the goal of finding very well ripened seeds. Take off the very fine tissue that covers them, leaving them completely white. Then grind or pulverize them in order to obtain a liquid containing finely divided solids in suspension, which must be mixed with a hundred grams of pure water. We must perform this procedure the night before the day that we intend to drink it. This must be done in order to leave it in repose for approximately ten or twelve hours.

In the morning hours, before drinking the beverage, it must be warmed in a double boiler. After drinking it, it is advisable to drink a little bit of heated water with the sole purpose of taking away the bad taste from our mouth.

This marvelous and magical beverage must be taken daily until one feels cured.

Calculi, Hepatic: Formula to Eject the Hepatic Calculi (Stones) without Surgical Operation

INGREDIENTS:
"Cholagogue" on branch	
"Cadillo de perro" or "cadillo mono"	
Nettle	
Glauber salts	3 ounces
Epsom salts	3 ounces

Boil these plants in three liters of water, leaving this decoction until the water is reduced to half. Once this preparation has cooled, then add the salts.

The ritual that has to be performed with the elementals of these plants is indispensable.

Calculi, Hepatic (Hepatic Stones) Olive oil and lemon

A) Consume half a glass of olive oil before going to sleep and another equal quantity in the morning on an empty stomach. Then, take a purgative of magnesium or salts, etc.

Consume a quantity of garlic within rum, etc.

B) Consume half a glass of olive oil mixed with the juice of several lemons. This has to be performed twice: consume one dosage before going to sleep and the other when you get up in the morning.

After the second dose of olive oil mixed with lemon, the patient will purge himself. The purgative must be done with magnesium or epsom salts or resin oil. A small bottle of castor oil or resin oil is preferable.

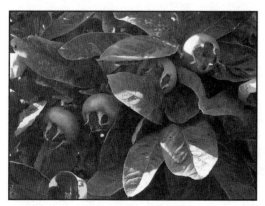

MEDLAR

Thus, the hepatic calculi (stones) will be ejected.

Calculi, Hepatic (Stones)

Place half a kilo of hen's gizzards within a bottle of white wine. Use the skin—that is to say, the thin skin of the gizzard—very well cleaned without scraping it.

This will be left to macerate for twenty days within the sweet white wine. After the twentieth day, the patient will consume one cup upon getting up in the morning, for nine days. After the ninth day, the patient will purge himself, consuming a small bottle of resin oil. Thus, he will eject the calculi.

Calculi (Stones): Formula to Eject from the Kidneys

With a lot of faith, the patient will consume a little cup of warm olive oil and lemon juice, and then a chamomile tea. Consume the whole of this remedy in the morning upon awakening, then afterwards lie down on the side of your liver (right side).

Cancer

What is cancer...? We answer this question by emphasizing the idea that it is the disorderly and anarchical development of cells in the patient's own organism. Is cancer contagious? The scientific experiments performed in the Institute for Experimental Medicine of Argentina were conclusive. The scientists placed sick rats and healthy rats together in the same cage. Unquestionably, they did not discover any type of contagion. Rats of different sexes were placed within such properly controlled experiments and were found without contagion. In the scientific world, it has been stated that rats that were fed with cancerous tumors did not become infected. They affirm that rats that were injected with the blood of a sick animal remained immune, without contagion.

Can any type of wound cause cancer? This type of question has an extraordinary importance from the civil and legal points of view, because of the claims that could be made for compensation of work accidents. These claims could be attributed as causes of cancer that any given employee can acquire from a work injury. It is clear that little wounds frequently repeated in the same place could be the cause of this terrible sickness, yet for only one wound, even if it is a strong wound, the answer is a decisive NO.

For this intelligent scientific conclusion, what was taken into account were the bullet wounds produced during the First World War of 1914-1918.

Does a germ produce cancer? Official science affirms that no, it does not. They emphasize the concept that this frightful sickness is not caused by any type of microbe or germ.

Revolutionary, scientific Gnosticism permits itself, with all respect, the liberty of disagreeing. We, the Gnostics, affirm the existence of the "**cancro**," the microbe or germ of cancer.

Is cancer transmittable? It is obvious that after many experiments, official science answers with a categorical NO. Nevertheless, exceptions do exist; for example: cancer was inoculated into a rat that was nourished with a diet poor in copper and low in catalase. The result was positive;

the rat became infected. It is indubitable that always when this experiment has been repeated, the same results have been obtained.

In another experiment, cancer was inoculated into a rat that had been previously prepared with a diet very rich in copper and catalase. The result was negative; the rat was not infected. Official science has discovered that hydrogen peroxide, "oxygenated water," particularly increases the catalase and protects against the undesirable development of cancer.

We understand that the germ of cancer, the terrible "cancro," is developed within organisms that are deficient in copper and catalase. It is unquestionable that the "cancro" cannot be seen, not even through the most potent electro-microscopes. However, if this dreadful sickness can be transmitted to organisms that are poor in copper and catalase, then it is obvious that such a microbe does exist.

The cancer germ itself develops and unfolds within the fourth dimension. It only allows itself to be observed in the tri-dimensional world through its destructive effects.

Undoubtedly, a very powerful electro-microscope will be invented in the future. Then, the "cancro" will be perceptible to the ultra-modern scientists.

It is clear that this fatal germ arrives to the planet Earth submerged within electromagnetic currents from the constellation of Cancer. By all means, cancer is the karma of fornication. It is obvious that ancient wise men knew in depth this very special type of nemesis.

Here in Mexico, there is a very special plant that can cure cancer. I want to emphatically refer to a certain bush-plant that is known in the region of Ixmiquilpan,

state of Idalgo. The name of this bush-plant is "aranto." Ancient aboriginal people baptized this plant with the indigenous name of "aulaga."

The complete data, which is delivered by our beloved Gnostic brother Alfonso Silva, is very interesting.

"Mr. Mario Aponte, chief of the office of the former Electric Force and Light Company from the Mexican Republic, Misquiahuala, Idalgo, was attacked by a sickness in his gums. It is obvious that he did not acknowledge it. He then traveled to Mexico City with the good purpose of consulting the physicians from the electricians' union. They diagnosed him with cancer of the mouth.

"Unsatisfied with such a diagnosis, the mentioned gentleman consulted with other doctors. However, the diagnosis given by all of them was the same.

"Mr. Aponte returned to Misquiahuala very afflicted. Obviously, he could not remain absent from his office for a long time.

"This cited gentleman narrated that a little old lady from that region made a commitment to heal him with a vegetal tea, which she herself would give him to drink in her presence. This was because she feared the patient would not drink the remedy on his own.

"The results were extraordinary. In the period of eight months, Mr. Aponte was radically cured.

"He continued drinking the old lady's tea. It was not necessary for her to give him the tea or to beg him to drink it, because the cited man asked for it daily.

"One month later, the doctors of Mexico City had to acknowledge with astonishment that the cancer had disappeared."

The Gnostic brother Alfonso Silva continued by saying:

"To this date, among all the people to whom I have offered the aranto or aulaga, I remember the name of Mrs. Luisa Lara de Barroeta, who is my sister-in-law. She was near to being operated on within the Social Security Institute for a cancerous tumor. It was the type of tumor in the womb, something very grave.

"This sick woman became radically healed by drinking infusions of aranto, and to this day she lives totally cured."

Thus, our Frater Silva continues by telling us the following:

"Mr. Agustin Uribe's spouse (we do not wish to reveal her address) was prepared by physicians to have a tumor from her liver extracted. Yet, when they verified that this was a cancerous tumor, they immediately stitched her up, obviously declaring her a lost case. She had no chance since the doctors found her abdominal cavity filled with cancerous tumors.

"However, this sick woman was definitively healed with the aranto and still lives thanks to the astonishing virtues of this bush-plant."

The distinguished physician, Doctor of Medicine Jacinto Juarez Parra from the National University of Mexico, tested the power of this bush-plant on a cancerous, terminally ill woman, already without hope. In this case it was indeed very difficult and not possible to save the life of this sick woman. I think that when the organism is already totally destroyed because of this sickness, every remedy fails.

Dr. Juarez considers that research with the electronic microscope can and must be performed on this whole plant. By centrifugation, the nucleus, the lysosomes, the ribosomes, and the microsomes must be separated in order to make a spectro-photometric analysis of each one of the parts of this plant. This would be for the intelligent purpose of discovering its colloids, enzymes, and its print or oligo element.

It must be investigated, says Dr. Juarez, to see which intracellular portions of this cited plant effectively act over the cancer. The mentioned physician continues saying that every cancerous patient, who is diagnosed through stimulating cytology and biopsy, will be medicated with the "Aranto," as well as dosages of catalase and copper, and later he will again make another measurement with the diagnostic data. Catalase and copper are low in cancerous people, and this has already been completely demonstrated. It is necessary to investigate the amount of sanguineous catalase and the dosage of copper in the plasma. Any organism poor in catalase and copper is a proper field for the complete development of the dreadful "cancro."

It has been broadcasted that the pseudo-sapient scientists offer hundreds of millions of dollars to the person who can deliver to them an effective formula that will cure cancer. The great multimillionaire Rockefeller has offered his ultra-modern laboratories to those who wish to experiment in the department of cancer research. The power of healing is not obtained with money and this is the failure of therapeutics for the determined and deadly sicknesses of this day and age.

Radium (chemotherapy) does not cure cancer. The radium waves burn the living cells, and if indeed a regression of the evolving process of the sickness is obtained, the cancer re-appears much later with yet more violence. Thus, the victim irremediably dies.

Through me, the venerable White Lodge freely delivers to humanity the infallible formula in order to cure cancer. Moreover, it despises the filth of money and for the same reason rejects the offered retribution. The formula is as follows:

Rum (alcoholic beverage) must be poured within a mate gourd (the fruit of the mate gourd with its pulp comes from a tree found in the hot regions of Colombia, and is often used by the peasants as utensils for the kitchen), along with mineral charcoal, "paraguay" (*Scoparia dulcis, L.*, a plant that is found in mild climates and is also called "escudilla," similar to the wormseed plant), and lemon. The whole of this is left to macerate for fifteen days. Then, the patient should drink it by little cupfuls, one every hour.

Bathe the body with a decoction of the leaves and roots from the apricot tree. During the bath, pronounce the mantra "**Rotando**" as you drink the medicine, like this:

> *Roooooooooooooo*
> *Taaaaaaaannnnnnnnnnnnn*
> *Doooooooooooooooooooo*

Before collecting the plants that are in the composition of this formula, one must walk in a circle, from right to left, from south to north, around each one of the plants, and while performing this, one must beg each of the elementals to heal the cancer.

Afterwards, the plants are caressed, blessed, and then collected. When the components are within the mate gourd, the mantra "Rotando" must be pronounced as we already explained. Then, with all the might of our willpower, the elementals of the plants must be commanded in order to heal the sick person.

The elementals are the life of the plants. Only life can fight against sickness and death. The seminal force of the plants are the instrument of the elementals.

Cancer, External

For the external cancerous ulcer.

Phenolic acid	quarter of an ounce
Camphor	half of a gram
Crystallized menthol	20 centigrams
Nitric acid	quarter of an ounce

Gently brush this on the cancerous ulcer three times a day and apply the following pomade:

Simple vaseline	
Permanganate	
Tincture of iodine	5 to 7 drops
Crystallized menthol	
Phenolic acid	3 to 5 drops
Starch	

The external cancer will disappear with this treatment.

Second Procedure to Cure Cancer

Finally, after many investigations and painful battles, we have discovered the marvelous and very efficacious plant that radically cures cancer. We can say goodbye to cancer with this plant that is within our reach.

The mentioned plant is the "ojaransin." Let the research of this plant be performed by those demented people, those who oppose the wisdom of Nature and who believe they have everything within their laboratories. Those false scientists (who abdicate reason because they derive their observations and knowledge from the microscope), arrive at boastful conclusions with a good amount of money in their pockets.

Well then, this important plant that we are occupying ourselves with, the "ojaransin," must be boiled in order to use in baths and in beverages.

This plant is very common in the state of Bolivar, Colombia. It grows in swampy areas. It is small in size, with lanceolate leaves, some of them possessing grayish points.

This plant also grows by the shores of rivers. Its name is indigenous. It is very well known by the Indians (the Majaguas), who inhabit the regions that are close to the community of Majagual (which is situated between the rivers San Jorge and Cauca, at the foot of Mojana's Jet, north of Sierra Ayapel, south of the state of Bolivar and bordered with Antioquia).

Upon their indigenous altars, the Majagua Indians hold this plant as a very sacred item. They utilize the elemental of this plant for important works of practical magic. This vegetal elemental looks like a completely naked child of some 20 centimeters in height. His two eyes look like two lanterns.

For Cancer

The rattlesnake cures cancer. The rattles and the head of the snake are eliminated (these parts are useless); the skin can be taken off. The meat is then dried under the sun, or at low heat (in the kitchen); when the meat is dried, it should be crushed and ground to a fine powder. Pour this substance into empty capsules in order to consume it. Take these capsules every two or three hours, in accordance with the sickness, and decrease the amount of capsules until eradicating this illness. Do not eat any type of meat.

ANOTHER FORMULA:

Cut off the rattles and the head of the snake. Set the meat out to dry under the sun. Once the meat is dry, pulverize it. Then, consume one spoonful of this powder mixed with three spoonfuls of olive oil,

two times a day. If the cancer is external, then the powder must be applied to the sick part.

Testimony about Cancer

After having delivered the formula of the rattlesnake, the number of people who have been cured from cancer can be counted by the thousands.

Ninety-nine percent of the cancer patients have been healed by means of the rattlesnake.

Therefore, the Gnostic medics have triumphed. Yet, the doctors of official science have not triumphed due to the following factors.

1. Incredibility and skepticism.

2. The tendency of administering other aids, other remedies, other medications to the patient.

It is obvious that the rattlesnake remedy is extremely jealous. If another remedy is administered to the cancer patient, the marvelous therapeutic effect of the rattlesnake is completely destroyed.

Moreover, one must know how to administer this remedy to the patient.

Head and rattles must be removed from the serpent. Only the meat of its trunk (which must be reduced to a powder) can be utilized in order to heal the patient.

It is clear that in order to cure the poor cancer patient, the powder of the pulverized meat must be put into capsules.

DOSAGE: One large capsule every hour.

Consecutively consume this remedy until the cancer is totally cured.

Any other remedy is absolutely prohibited. Not even analgesics like aspirin, etc., are accepted, because otherwise the curative power of the rattlesnake is lost.

In the name of truth, I emphatically affirm that cancer is no longer a problem.

Cancer is a problem for the "foolish scientists" of this frightful age of the Antichrist, but never for the Gnostic medics who work with the rattlesnake.

Cataract of the Eyes

The efficiency of this formula sets it apart from other similar ones.

At high tide, obtain a young "hobo" plant (*spondias purpurea l.*). Cut a thick stalk, which must then be peeled, scraped and its leaves taken off. Next, cut it into pieces that are about twenty centimeters long, more or less. With your mouth, blow into the circular stalk so that the air pressure will push the sap out of it. Collect this sap in a jar, then dampen a chamomile branch with this liquid. Apply these drops into the eyes of the sick person. It is important to take into account that the drops must flow down from the chamomile branch.

The "hobo" is a leafy and tall tree from the "terebintaceas" species. Its fruit is similar to the plum.

Cataract or Fleshiness in the Eyes

Put green rue (*ruta graveolens l.*), chamomile, flowers and plantain leaves (*plantago major l.*) into an amber colored jar or a white one if an amber colored one is not available. Once these plants are within the jar, put it under the sun from eight in the morning until five in the afternoon. When you get up in the morning put two drops in each eye. You must buy Collyrium Furancin Ophthalmic Solution in order to put two drops of this solution in each eye (one hour after putting in the first drops). Do this three times a day.

Against Catarrh

This tormenting sickness is easy to cure.

Every morning, filled with a lot of faith, consume half an ounce of sugar on an empty stomach.

It is advisable to consume rhubarb every week. It is enough to put a spoonful of rhubarb powder into boiling water. Consume a glass of it before dinner. This dose of rhubarb needs to be taken only once a week. This is a marvelous remedy for catarrh.

Chancres

Apply "aristol" and "juan" powders on the chancres.

Chilblains

In order to radically cure chilblains, the area must be washed daily, with a great deal of patience within a very hot decoction of turnip roots.

Children Who Lose Their Appetite and Have Fetid Defecation

One leaf of wormwood (*artemisia absinthium*), three grams of fennel (*foeniculum vulgare mill.*), Three grams of chamomile (*Anthemis nobilis L.*): boil all of these in water. Lactose must be added plus 3 drops of "Vi-penta" (from the pharmacy). Consume twice a day.

Chlorosis (see also Dropsy)

This terrible sickness is very frequent in children and also abounds among adults. The sick person becomes swollen and the blood rapidly impoverishes itself. The internal organs do not work properly, and exhaustion with its innumerable consequences produces a perennial martyrdom.

Bathe the sick person with warm water and earth soap, pine soap, or with whatever soap is at hand. Then, suspend this bath and immediately after, bathe with:

Water	6 liters
Kitchen salt	2 ounces
Glauder salts	2 ounces
Iodine	1/2 ounce

Frequently apply intestinal cleanses with Sen of Castile. Bottle up the following formulae into two bottles. Give the patient one small cup of the formula from bottle number one before each meal and another small cup from bottle number two after each meal.

Formula One:

Boldo's extract	1/2 ounce
Quina's extract	1/2 ounce
Tincture of nux vomica	30 drops
Rhubarb's extract	1/2 ounce
Quinine	1/2 gram
Caffeine	1/2 gram
Tincture of aconite	30 drops

Formula Two:

Water	1 liter
"Vichi" salts	1 spoonful
Cream of tartar	1 ounce
Citric acid	1 ounce

Cirrhosis

Formula:	
"Tatua" plant	1 pound
Panela (hard sugar cane)	1 panela
Glauber salts	1 ounce
Epsom salts	1 ounce

Once the ritual of the tatua plant is performed, its leaves must then be collected. Make sure to detach the leaves starting from top to bottom. If the leaves are collected in the opposite manner (from bottom to top) it will produce vomiting.

Parboil the "tatua" plant; when the water is boiling add the panela. Reduce the fire, let it repose and then bottle it up. Take one spoonful every hour.

Colic (Hepatic Colic)

In order to cure women's hepatic colic, male goat manure will be utilized. The male goat manure must be dissolved in cold water. It should then be strained and boiled. It must be taken every other day until three active days are completed.

For men, the case is similar, the difference being that the manure must be from a female goat.

Conjunctivitis

The decoction of the leaves of the plant called "prosopis," "ñandubay" (which is very abundant in the Argentinean territory) is good for conjunctivitis.

After having filtered the decoction very well, one must employ it for ocular washing in the evident cases of conjunctivitis.

This plant is marvelous. The patient will wash his eyes; he has to put the water from the decoction of this plant into a good container. Then, he has to immerse his wide opened eyes within this water. This is the way to wash the eyes.

This remedy must be performed daily until one is healed.

Constipation

Constipation must be combated with teas of chicory with lemon, or teas of plums, flax, rhubarb (*rheum spp.*), agar agar (*gelidium cartilagineum*), boxwood (*buxus sempervirens l.*), cascara sagrada (*rhamnus purshiana dc.*), chard, orange juice, etc.

One teaspoon daily of castor oil on an empty stomach helps to eliminate constipation.

Constipation

Three prunes, one liter of unsweetened water: drink it before meals.

This is very good for children, however the quantity must be reduced.

Corns

For those tormenting corns on the hands and fingers: dab them with silver nitrate.

Cough

Any cough, as bothersome as it may be, can be cured with teas made from following plants:

Eucalyptus, milkwort (*polygala vulgaris*), horehound (*marrubium vulgare l.*), coltsfoot (*tussilago farfara*), maidenhair fern (*adiantum capillus-veneris l.*), "anacahuita," "ambay," "drosera," "scabious," "chachacoma" (*escallonia tubar mutis*).

Cough, Remedy for Various Types of Chest Coughs

Chicory, celery, and eucalyptus: consume the decoction four times a day.

Cough, Adult

Decoction of the following plants: eucalyptus and fragrant pine. This can be consumed at night, before going to sleep, with or without sweetener. This recipe serves to take away that rebellious cough that could not be taken away with any other type of expectorant.

Cough, Bronchial

Bronchial coughs are cured with the root of licorice, sweetroot, "regaliz."

Boil a good quantity of the root of licorice and drink this tea as an ordinary beverage until becoming healed.

The Gnostic medics must never forget the rituals or magic works with the elementals of the plants.

Cough, Bronchitis; Chronic Asthma

Besides helping coughs, bronchitis, asthma, obesity, etc., horehound (*marrubium vulgare l.*) is also useful against lack of appetite and other digestion disorders in general.

A medicinal wine can be prepared with twenty grams of horehound. It is enough to leave the twenty grams of this plant in maceration within a bottle of wine.

This maceration must endure for forty days. One little cupful of this medicine, as an appetizer, will be consumed before every meal.

Cough, Children

A remedy for a cough that harasses children too much is the following: take honey (bee honey) and squeeze one lemon into it, then add a little bit of sulphur. Give this to them in small spoonfuls.

Also, here is another worthy remedy: squeeze out the juice of one lemon and make sugared-honey (make it with sugar). Have the child swallow this.

Cough, Children; Another Recipe

Decoction of five grams of borage (*borago officinalis l.*), "tusiago" or any expectorant, and a quarter of a bromoquinine tablet. In the beginning, it has to be consumed twice a day, and later on, only once a day. This remedy takes the cough away from children.

Croup

TREATMENT: The sick person must gargle with the decoction of rice, vinegar, and barley.

Deafness

Bathe the ear internally and externally with honey (bee honey), thus the deafness will disappear. (EDITOR: see also RATTLESNAKE MEDICATIONS, pg. 159).

Diabetes

After having blessed the following plants (as is performed in all cases), collect the leaves of avocado tree, the leaves of walnut tree, and the leaves of eucalyptus tree. Boil these leaves and give the patient three glasses to drink daily (one before each meal). It is important to note that the first morning portion is taken on an empty stomach.

ANOTHER FORMULA: Bark from myrtle, bark from mango, "volsamina."

Diabetes

The honey-water extracted from the trunk of the maguey (*agave americana l.*) serves also to cure diabetes. For one year, consume three glassfuls daily, one before each meal.

Diabetes

Thirty grams of "pedralejo" or "chaparro" with ten grams of eucalyptus or walnut, three times a day.

Diabetes

Eliminating anger and the inferior emotions, anxieties, and violent acts cures diabetes. Also, drink teas or decoctions from the plant called in Mexico "lagrimas de san pedro" (*coix lacryma-jobi l.*).

Diabetes

Diabetes is deadly, yet by swallowing bull's gall bile the patient can be cured.

Whosoever wants to be cured of the horrible diabetes must eliminate from within the undesirable psychic elements of anger, preoccupation, anxieties, sadness, fear, and anguish. These psychological defects alter the nervous system. An altered nervous system destroys the pancreas and produces diabetes.

Diabetes

Another remedy to cure diabetes that is less horrible than the bull's gall bile is the following:

Collect some river crabs, dry them as best as you can within an oven, then reduce them to a very fine powder.

Then, add sugar to these powders, but only a very little bit of sugar; remember that you have diabetes. Afterwards, put a little bit of iron water in this preparation.

The iron water is not a problem to make. To make the iron water, place iron filings that you will use within the water. You can find iron filings in any blacksmith's shop.

Diabetes

The diabetic person who wants to be cured must eliminate anger, preoccupation, anguish, fear, etc. from his psyche.

Diabetes

There are many plants to cure diabetes; some of these plants may be more favorable than others for the sick person.

Different teas can be drunk such as: wild celery (*apium graveolens l.*), "sarandil blanco," black mulberry, walnut, "pesuña de vaca," watercress, artichoke or wild artichoke, "lagrimas de san pedro" (*coix lacryma-jobi l.*), etc.

Anti-diabetic Tea

The following anti-diabetic tea must be prepared with a bunch of "pesuña de vaca" leaves, any quantity of leaves of wild celery, a bunch of black mulberry tree leaves, a good quantity of dandelion leaves, and a bunch of "sarandil blanco" leaves.

All of these leaves must be very well boiled in water. Use a pot of water in order to boil them and drink it as an ordinary beverage for your thirst.

If some of these plants cannot be obtained, the anti-diabetic tea can be prepared with the remaining plants.

In accordance with elementotherapy, the plants must be blessed and the elementals must be commanded to cure the pancreas.

This tea must be drunk daily (without ever getting tired of drinking it) until one is healed.

Diabetes, Intestinal Inflammation, Gases, Indigestion, Burps, Etc.

The plant called "marcela" (*Alternanthera ramosissima Chodat*) cures diabetes as well as bothersome burps, gas, and indigestion, etc. Boil thirty grams of the flowers of this plant and consume this tea.

Dosage: Three glassfuls daily, one after each meal. This tea must be drunk daily until one becomes totally healed.

Diabetes, Unrestrained Urine, Pain and Swelling of the Breasts of Mothers Who Are Breast Feeding

There is a remedy, which is apparently very repugnant, in order to cure diabetes, unrestrained urine, and all the sicknesses already cited in this part of the book.

I want to emphatically refer to mouse manure. There is no doubt that this manure cures these illnesses. It is important to consume one spoonful of this manure and to mix it with the pressed juice of the plant called plantain (*Plantago major L.*).

That mixture needs to be consumed or drunk in the morning on an empty stomach and upon going to sleep. The results will be marvelous.

In order to radically eliminate the swelling of the breast of breast-feeding mothers, it is enough to dissolve the powders of mouse manure within a little bit of natural water and to humidify the breasts with this marvelous water.

Diarrhea

There are many plants with which we can make teas to cure diarrhea. Let us remember rice, which is so healthful and marvelous. "Guarrus" can be prepared with it.

The hot teas of mallow (*malva sylvestris l.*), nettle (*urtica dioica l.*), or roses are marvelous to cure diarrhea.

Also helpful are the teas of knotgrass (*polygonum aviculare l.*), "tormentilla," pearl barley, the leaves of sour guava tree with lemon, well-cooked.

Diarrhea

When diarrhea is produced because of heat, consume the infusion of the root or the branch of lemongrass (*cymbopogon citratus*). When diarrhea is produced because of cold, then consume the infusion of cinnamon with peppermint.

Diarrhea

Any one of the diverse teas or decoctions of sweet basil (*ocimum basilicum l*), cañaigre (*rumex hymenosepalus torr.*), "chaparro amargoso," "suelda conselda" (*tradescantia multiflora swz.*), etc., make diarrhea disappear.

Diarrhea

The "Mama" Matias healed a strong case of diarrhea with water and ashes from the open fire used for cooking.

The ashes are mixed with water. Leave this mixture in repose for a while. Stir it again and give this mixture to the sick person to drink.

This formula never fails.

ANOTHER FORMULA:
Decoction of the root of Ipecacuana

	6 grams
Sulfate of sodium	20 grams
Syrup of cinnamon	30 grams

This must be drunk, very well mixed, in little cupfuls.

ANOTHER FORMULA: Leaves of "tuatua" (*jatropha gossypifolia l.*), which must be collected by detaching them from bottom up (starting from the bottom and continuing up until reaching the top) and shoots of "uvito."

Diarrhea, Very Grave

FORMULA:
Roots of pomegranate
Chamomile
Internal thin skin of a hen's gizzards

Bless the plants as usual, and cook everything. Consume the decoction by little cupfuls. This remedy never fails. It is infallible.

FORMULA TWO: A small handful of leaves from the coca plant boiled in water or in milk will be enough to heal the sick person in the very act of drinking this decoction.

Against Bad Digestion

There is marvelous formula to aid bad digestion.

FORMULA:

Anise	four ounces
Fennel	four ounces
Coriander	half an ounce
Powdered licorice	half an ounce
One ground nutmeg	
Cinnamon	a good quantity
Sugar	a small spoonful

Mix all of these elements and put the medicine into a jar. One small spoonful of this powder must be consumed at the end of every meal.

Bad Digestion and Intestinal Disorders

Perform intestinal cleansings (enemas) with the decoction of mallow (*malva sylvestris l.*) and sweet basil (*ocimum basilicum*) plants. Also, drink three glassfuls daily, one before each meal.

One daily intestinal cleansings (enema) with mallow is how the patient will become healed.

Bad Digestion

In Chile, there is a plant called "mallico." This vegetal is formidable in order to combat bad digestion.

Use thirty grams of the root of this plant per one liter of water. Boil it very well.

Drink a large glassful after each meal.

Digestion, Difficult

When digestion is difficult, then it is convenient to drink teas from any one of the following plants: "prodigiosa," rosemary, "tabaquillo grande," "indian" tea, "ranchero" tea, castilleja spp., "yolochichi." The sick person can and must prepare his beverages with any of the aforementioned plants that could be found.

Diphtheria

Water, boric acid, citrate of potassium (for gargling).

Dropsy

The decoction of guaiacum (*guaiacum officinale l.*) cures dropsy. One must drink three glassfuls daily, one before each meal, until becoming radically healed.

Dropsy

The flowers of "maravilla bastarda," which is the wild four-o-clock plant (*mirabilis multiflora torr.*), is magnificent for dropsy.

Put a bunch of these flowers within a glass of white wine (it is advisable to do this between the hours of six in the afternoon and six in the morning).

You must place the container that holds this marvelous magic infusion over the ashes of hot charcoal.

The sick person will drink from this liquid and then consume a very concentrated broth of beef soup.

This remedy will be taken for eight days. The magical ritual of elementotherapy must be performed with the flowers so that the elementals will heal the sick person.

Dysentery

We cannot deny that "emetina" in ampoules heals dysentery. However, children must not be injected with "emetina" because they will die. Nonetheless, there are marvelous plants that cure dysentery. Let us look at the following:

Cotton, black or wild cherry (*prunus serotina ehrh.*), "chaparro amargoso," ipecac (*cephaelis ipecacuanha*), common plantain (*plantago major l.*), mesquite (*prosopis juliflora l.*), "monacillo" (*malvaviscus arboreus cav.*), "muicle" (*jacobinia spicigera [schl] b.*), "nanche," etc.

Any of these plants can cure dysentery. They must be drank as beverages, like drinking ordinary water, until one is healed.

Ear Infection (Pus)

Half a gram of carbolic acid within thirty grams of glycerin will be enough in order to apply this by drops in the ear.

Ear Itchiness

Put one or two drops of warmed glycerin in the ear at night.

Eczema, Dry or Purulent Rashes on the Extremities (Limbs, Hands, Feet) or on the Body

DECOCTION OF:
Gualanday (*jacaranda caucana pittier*)
                       thirty grams
"Grama blanca"   thirty grams
Bark of oak ("flor amarilla")   thirty grams
Horsetail (*equisetum arvense l.*)
Sarsaparilla (the root, *smilax officinalis*)

The following plants are used in order to bathe the affected parts: "frutillo" (big leaves, *rauvolfia ligustrina roem.*) and "matandrea" (*alpinia occidentalis*) or from plums (coast of Colombia).

FORMULA FOR AN OINTMENT FOR ECZEMA: Add sulphur to one ounce of "otova" (nutmeg of Colombia) and 25 drops of phenolic acid, 5 drops of "canime." Mix everything together and dab this cream upon the affected area at night before going to bed and after bathing the affected area.

In addition to drinking three glassfuls daily of the decoction above (of five aforementioned plants), the patient must also alternately drink "amargo sulphuroso y tricocalcio" (bitter sulphuric and tricocalcium), a remedy that contains three types of limes—mineral, vegetal, and animal—must be drank. First, consume the bitter one, then the calcium; at least three small bottles or jars of each one.

No type of meat can be eaten during the treatment, nor should one drink any type of liquor. Absolutely no liquor or meat should be consumed.

Elephantiasis

Drinking the water within which there was previously an elephant cures elephantiasis. The person must even wash his body with this water.

Elephantiasis, Swellings, and Ulcers

Swellings and ulcers afflicting people who suffer from elephantiasis are healed with the oil within which a viper had been placed under the sun. Every day the sick person will wash his face and his scabs or ulcers with the water (within which a snake had been placed).

Epilepsy

Senobarbital is a remedy sold in pharmacies. Give the patient burnt rinds of sour orange: grind them first and then give it to him. The patient should not drink coffee or liquor.

Epileptic Illness or Epilepsy of the Heart

Even though it seems incredible, when turkey manure is dissolved in wine or in plantain (*plantago major L.*) water, it is completely proven that it cures the horrible epileptic illness or epilepsy of the heart. Consume it continuously until becoming healed.

Epilepsy, Nervous
(See also PARTURIENT WOMEN, CRAZINESS OF, and EPILEPSY BECAUSE OF COLDNESS IN THE OVARIES)

Take a spoonful each hour of the following formula:

Camphorated water	1 bottle
Bromide of potassium	1 gram
Bromide of ammoniac	1 gram
Bicarbonate of potassium	half of an ounce
Tincture of calabar bean	2 ounces
Tincture of belladonna	2 ounces

An abundant amount has been written about epilepsy, yet the adequate remedy in order to cure this sickness has yet to be discovered. Generally, it is accepted that the possessed people referred to in the sacred scriptures were simply epileptic people. Indeed, they were epileptic. However, larvae or demons from the submerged worlds possessed them.

In the third paragraph of page 111 of the novel *Rosy Cross*, by the Master Krumm-Heller (Huiracocha), Argentinean edition, we read:

> "Saint Alphonse who is cited by Padre Neyraguet in his Compendium of Theology says: Contra malefitia utilicet remedis ex medicina petitis plures enimverba ut ruta, et salvia, etcetera, contra malifitia naturalites prosunt, quia virtute naturali, corrigunt pravos umeros ope demonis comotos. Articulis IV, De Maleficio, Perrone dice: Nihil eni, vetat quominus dicamus interdum qui a cloemace agitabantur aut amentia, aut epilepsia laborare cum et hin morbi a cloemone ipso injice posunt. Deo ita permittente, uti plures pres ac interpretes censure."

Sage (*salvia officinalis l.*) and rue (*ruta graveolens l.*) are the magic plants that the Gnostic medic utilizes in order to cure people who are possessed by demons (epileptic people).

The procedure with the sage plant is as follows: The plant is harvested at night, so that after it is blessed, it is yanked by surprise from its very roots. The pressed juice (obtained by scrubbing the leaves in water) is given to the patient to drink. This plant's smoke can also be used for smudging (fumigating). The sick person must be directly smudged with the smoke. This is done in combination with prayer, in which the medic magician has to be filled with faith.

In ancient times, an accessory, made with long pieces of glass, was used for smudging, in combination with an exorcism from a secret book. In this day and age, the CONJURATION OF THE FOUR can be utilized, as it appears in the chapter entitled, "Cases of Psychic Possession" (pages 52-55). Everything that is mentioned there must be taken into account in order to cure epileptic people.

The elemental of the sage plant has a pale yellow colored tunic and has the power of healing possessed people. The rue's smoke will be employed along with the smoke of the sage plant.

Epilepsy; Magic Procedure in Order to Cure

This frightful sickness is karmic and it is due to the fact that the patient was dedicated to Spiritism or Spiritualism (as it is called here in Mexico) in his former lives.

Obviously, the epileptic person was a medium of Spiritism. Therefore, it is not irrelevant to emphatically affirm that the Karma, which the mediums of Spiritism originate, is that which is called "epilepsy."

Obviously, epileptic people are possessed by tenebrous entities from the inferior regions of the Astral Plane.

MAGIC FORMULA

Sit the epileptic person within a refreshing and pleasant garden. Then, recite in his ear the following magical words:

Oremus Preceptis Salutaris Monitis

Afterwards, you must pray the "Pater Noster," which is "The Lord's Prayer."

This work must be performed daily.

If helping the sick person is what is wanted, then, the linden tree (*tilia spp.*) can also be used.

An incision in the trunk of this tree must be done in the month of February. The water that pours out from the trunk of this tree can be given to the patient to drink.

DOSAGE: Three ounces of this water each week. This is how epileptic people can be cured.

The Gnostic medic must not forget to perform the magic circle around the linden tree.

The supplication to the elemental of the Linden tree must not be forgotten as well. Thus, that elemental creature can cure the epileptic person.

Erysipelas

The aloe vera, famous for its multiple properties, is a powerful remedy and without equal for the healing of erysipelas. Once it is baked, it is enough to rub it over the affected area.

Another effective remedy is the preparation of chameleon in powder with firewater. For such an operation, it is enough to rub the sick area with it. The toad produces similar effects when rubbing it over the affected area.

Erysipelas, Sores, Damage to the Skin, Cutaneous Infections, etc.; Formula in Order to Cure

Dissolve the following within lightly sugared water which must have been previously boiled:

Cream (of tartar)	1 ounce
Rhubarb	1 ounce
Manna	1 ounce
Jalap	1 ounce
Lemon	1 ounce
Panela (hard sugar cane)	250 grams

Consume this preparation by the spoonfuls once every hour. In addition, the sick person must strike his affected area with a branch of a plant called "bicho largo," in Colombia (which must be humidified with urine that has been heated up by sunlight).

If one proceeds in accordance with the given instructions, we are sure of the absolute efficiency of this formula, in spite of the laughter and distrust of the "know-it-alls."

Erysipelas, Against; Special formula

The following formula that we give here deserves complete attention because it is absolutely effective against erysipelas.

Get a green calabash, or, if that is not available, a green "totumo" (*crescentia cujete l.*). Roast it lightly in the embers or in the smoking ashes. Then, extract the pulp, which must be applied with salt over the leg or the area affected by the erysipelas. This procedure must be administered as hot as can be tolerated.

Moreover, before applying the cataplasms from the pulp of the calabash or "totumo," the sick person must drink strong black coffee, which must contain five grams of quinine. It is also suggested that the sick person applies the leaves of "matandrea" (alpina occidentalis) over the affected area (once the cataplasm is removed)

Erysipelas, Nervous

> FORMULA:
> Water of camphor
> Bromide of potassium   1 gram
> Bromide of ammonia   1 gram
> Bicarbonate of potassium   1 gram
> Tincture of calabar bean   8 grams
> Tincture of belladonna   1 ounce

Mix all of these together and consume one spoonful each hour. In addition to this, apply the formula that is written on the pages entitled "Cases of Psychic Possession" (pgs. 52-55).

Eye Sight

Squeeze cashew fruit into a very well-cleaned glass container. Then, add one gram of boric acid and leave it undisturbed in a dark place to macerate for the space of fifteen days. Place a black cloth over it, so that it can be in darkness. Then, strain it and leave it undisturbed for another fifteen days in the same dark place. When one month has passed (after the second fifteen days), then filter or strain it again. Put two drops daily in your eyes in the morning. This will increase the sight.

Eye Sight, Remedy in Order to Strengthen the Sight

The sunflower plant is very interesting, since it always orientates its flower towards the King Star (the Sun).

Whosoever wants to fortify his sight has to distill the leaves of the sunflower within very pure water.

Small, little cloths, very well cleaned and previously disinfected within boiling water, must be humidified with this water.

Thus, the cloths will be humidified within that distilled sunflower water when being absolutely sure that those cloths are clean.

It is clear that in accordance with the elementotherapy explained in this book, the ritual to the elemental of the sunflower must be performed, so that the elemental of that plant will cooperate in the healing and fortification of the eyes.

Eye Sty

Whosoever suffers from this stubborn affliction will be healed with the application of a freshly laid hen egg on the eye.

Fainting

Give the patient the plant called "destrabadora" (in Colombia) to smell. Also, the decoction of this plant must be given to the patient to drink. Do not forget the ritual of the plant.

Feet Inflammation

Dab the feet with camphorated oil and cover them with cotton.

Fevers, Common

(Read section regarding febrifuge plants, pg. 112)

Fever with Mad Disposition

(Read section regarding jarilla chivata, pg. 139)

Sulfate of quinine
Spearmint
Iodine   6 drops
"Creso"
Candle tallow
Kitchen salt

Join these ingredients and rub them on the body of the sick person, as many times as it is necessary.

Fever; To Cut Off Any Type

To a grated potato add pulverized marine "coha," and place this mixture over a piece of flannel, that is to say, enveloped by the flannel. Place this over the stomach. Put crushed green onions over the soles of the feet and hold them in place with a rag.

Old Fistulas

"Jarilla," "vira-vira," cortex of cinchona, sage, and "jarilla chivata."

Perform the ritual of the elementals of these plants. Then, boil them very well for

several hours. Make a cataplasm and apply it over the fistula.

Incurable Fistulas

Collect the roots of "guacamayo" (*protium heptaphyllum [l.] march.*) some that are facing the east and others that are facing west. These will be reduced to powder, and in such a manner they will be ready.

Now apply "piedralipe" with candle wax over the fistula and leave this mixture there for the space of twenty-four hours. Then, when this time is completed, proceed to wash the fistula and apply the powders of "guacamayo." The sick person can wait confidently, for his fistula will be healed.

Fistulas and Tinea

Even though it seems incredible (it is certain the proud intellectuals will not take advantage of this formula as well as other formulas contained in this book), we are going to present to you the following formula that gives astonishing results:

Urinate in a clean vessel. Then, mix ground common salt with your urine. Wash the fistula with this compound and then apply talcum over the fistula in order for it to become dry.

Fistulas, Rebel

The powders of the starch from purple "guaco" (*mikania guaco humb. & bonpl.*) applied over the fistulas produce excellent results.

Also the powders of oak when humidified with saliva and applied in the morning on an empty stomach give excellent results.

Fistulas or Ulcers

Plum tree: the water from its decoction serves marvelously in order to wash the fistulas or ulcers, especially those of the mouth.

Against Flatulence or Gas from the Bowels

This matter of abdominal gases, flatulence, or nauseating winds is extremely tormenting, and what is even worse is that they very greatly afflict the hemorrhoids. They can originate many tormenting illnesses.

It also happens that the gas from the bowels can rise unto the brain and damage it. For all of these reasons it is necessary to be cured.

The anise star (*illicium anisatum l.*) can be acquired in a plant market or in the pharmacies.

Drink the tea of this plant everyday in the morning when getting up from bed, until achieving the healing.

The Gnostic medics advise one infusion of this plant daily. This is how the sick person will become healed from this tormenting affliction.

Fractured Bones and Rheumatic Pains

Lion lard totally welds any bone. Therefore, osteopaths and massage therapists must use it. It also cures rheumatism.

The plant sansevieria (*sanseviera zeilanica*) must also be utilized by applying it as a cataplasm over the fractured or disarranged bones in order to heal them.

The center of the arm bone of the lion, when pulverized and drunk with rum gives an extraordinary agility to those who drink it.

Freckles or Spots on the Face

Take a mother-of-pearl shell and squeeze three lemons, until the shell is covered with the juice. If there are no shells available, then some mother-of-pearl buttons can be utilized. Leave this in maceration and after eight days a pomade will be formed. To every ounce of this pomade add twenty-five grams of borax or "atincar," nine grams of kitchen salt, and in order for this pomade to be enjoyable, add some perfume to it.

Wash the freckled area with warm water that contains nine grams of kitchen salt and nine grams of borax. Dry it very well and scrape the freckle, spot or scar with water-sandpaper, which is black in color, then dab the previously prepared pomade onto it. The next day clean it with a towel and dab cocoa butter on it during the night or during the day. Do not stay under the sun for the duration of this treatment.

Against the Horrible Freckles

Soak a little bit of cotton on a branch with hydrogen peroxide. Then, patiently, it will be applied during the space of five minutes over the freckles you wish to eliminate.

If the skin becomes irritated, wash it with boric acid dissolved at four percent.

Fungi

Fifteen grams of salicylic acid and seventy-five grams of alcohol.

Gangrene

Apply poultices with the decoction of the plant called stinkweed (*datura stramonium l.*)

Procedure: Boil the stinkweed in a new pot or container. Do not save the water that has already been used by the patient; the decoction must always be new. Cover the pot or container after emptying it. Destroy the pot when this remedy is no longer needed.

The stinkweed is a plant whose employment is very delicate.

Gas Pains

"Hipodespas," which is a pharmaceutical medicine, can be used for any part of the organism. It can be consumed in any dose required.

Gastralgia (Stomachache)

Whosoever proceeds to cure gastralgia with the following formula, will surely achieve it.

Magnesia calcite	4 grams
Rhubarb in powder	4 grams
Cinnamon in powder	4 grams

This compound must be mixed very well. It makes a total of twelve grams which should be evenly distributed and placed on twelve slips of paper; in other words, one gram for each slip of paper. Two of these must be consumed daily, one in the morning on an empty stomach, and the other at night. They must be consumed with a little bit of plain water.

Consuming one spoonful of horehound (*marrubium vulgare l.*) boiled with beer will cure it quickly.

Gastritis and Stomach Ulcers

It has already been demonstrated that the honey-water extracted from maguey (*agave americana l.*) becomes a marvelous beverage in order to cure gastritis and stomach ulcers.

Consume three glasses daily, one before each meal. We, the Mexicans, know very well what "pulque" is and from where it is extracted. Nonetheless, foreign people do not know anything about it; they do not even know what "pulque" is. So, we must explain that the honey-water is the base for the "pulque" and it can only be attained by pruning the maguey plant.

Gonorrhea

Formula number one:

Every morning, on an empty stomach, consume an egg yolk beaten in "canime" oil. Add sugar according to your taste. This treatment should be prolonged until being completely healed.

Formula number two:

Deposit nine fresh eggs into a glass jar, or if not available, a very well glazed pot. Then, squeeze a sufficient quantity of lemon juice to cover the eggs. Close the lid of the jar and leave the preparation sealed for ten days, because at the end of this period the lemon juice will have performed its purpose with the eggs. It is relevant to inform in advance that the eggs must be arranged without breaking them. Afterwards, the preparation has to be blended until the shells of the eggs have been reduced to fine grains (calcium). Then, it must be drained or filtered as best as possible, in order to pour a bottle of rum into it and sugar according to your taste. Bottle it up and drink it in little cupfuls three times a day. There are those whose state of weakness is so great, that only one dose is enough for them to pass out. Therefore, it is necessary for such people to decrease their dosage, which will be gradually increased until they can drink the full amount.

We also recommend this restorative drink for people with malaria, anemia, convalescence, etc.

Continuing, we cite a case that occurred in the city of Armenia (Quindio): Mr. M.S., twenty-two years of age, was suffering from gonorrhea for a period of four years. Distinct doctors, who were administering great dosages of penicillin, attended him. However, the sickness was continuing its course and causing harm to the poor, young organism of this wretched man, who as a last resort had thought of committing suicide. Fortunately, he had the opportunity to submit himself to formula number two (previously described), which was not slow in showing him improvements and sudden radical healing. Thus, in the eight years that followed, this cited man has not shown any signs of this terrible sickness again.

Gonorrhea, Artificial

There are sorcerers who know how to give artificial gonorrhea to their hated enemies. When this occurs, the official doctors definitely fail and the sick person suffers without relief.

This type of gonorrhea is cured with the decoction of little purslane ("verdolaguita"), mistletoe from the evergreen oak ("muerdago de encina"), and wild radish. Drink it daily.

Gonorrhea, Chronic

There are some people who think that chronic gonorrhea can be cured with penicillin. Really, penicillin serves to kill the incipient gonococci, that is to say, when the sickness is not chronic. If the sickness is chronic, the symptoms can cease with penicillin, the illness can be cut. However, afterwards the sickness returns with even more strength. That is all.

We offer the following formula in order to cure such gonorrhea.

Obtain branches of arnica (*arnica montana*), root of caesar weed (*urera baccifera [l.] gaud.*) little purslane ("verdolaguita"), "pito morreal," "bretonica," the root of maguey (*agave americana l.*), gualanday (*jacaranda caucana pittier*) and sarsaparilla (*smilax officinalis*). If all of these plants cannot be obtained, then the majority of them will be enough. Having all of them would be better, of course. It is necessary to never forget that plants are not the ones that cure, rather it is their elementals. Therefore, the magical rite must not be missing at the moment when harvesting these plants, precisely as we have already taught how to do.

Boil all of these plants for one hour. Three big glasses of this beverage must be drunk, one before each meal. In addition, the sick person must perform urethral washings with the following composition:

Boric acid	half an ounce
"Azucar plomo"	half an ounce
Sulfate of zinc	half an ounce
Boiled water	500 grams

Cleanse the liver, kidneys, spleen, stomach, and intestines with the following preparation:

Boiled water	1 liter
Glauber salts	3 ounces
Epsom salts	3 ounces
Tincture of rhubarb	1 ounce

Drink one little cupful in the morning on an empty stomach.

FORMULA:

Sulfate of alumine	2 grams
Sulfate of zinc	2 grams
Camphorated liquor	4 grams
Bee honey	15 grams
Distilled water	250 grams

This formula is for the performance of urethral baths, performed once daily.

Gonorrhea in Women

Juice from viche pineapple with sweet niter and sugar is effective for the cure of venereal diseases of the feminine sex.

Gonorrhea and Bladder Stones

Beat an egg yolk with "canime" oil and sugar. Take this remedy every day in the morning on an empty stomach.

Internal Wounds from Previous Gonorrhea

A case can occur in which a ray from the Moon produces an internal abscess with an inguinal (dried) infarction. When this occurs, a red line, that extends itself from the sexual glands down to the toes of the feet, necessarily appears.

In order to cure this illness, one must perform a sitz bath with the decoction of mulberry, laurel, "hoja de luna" leaf ("lulu," as it is named in the interior of Colombia), and stalk of sweet potato.

Goiter

Apply over the goiter a little plate of lead and leave it there for ninety days. This is enough in order for this inconvenient

sickness to totally disappear. Hence, the dangerous surgical operation is avoided, which in most cases always attracts fatal consequences.

Also, one can burn a natural sponge. As soon as it becomes like charcoal, it should be reduced to a fine powder. The sick person will drink one gram of this powder dissolved in half of a glass of water.

Salt mixed with saliva and applied over the goiter during the time of the waning moon also cures the goiter.

Gout; Gentle Purgative for Those Who Suffer

Make a decoction of willow (*salix alba l.*) after having ground it; then mix it with vinegar. Consume one spoonful in the morning for a period of nine days. This purgative will expel all of the thick tumors (which are an obstruction for the organism) from the stomach of the sick person.

Headaches, Chronic

Chronic headaches can be very easily cured: affix to the bottom of the feet of the patient the following:

Put oil and little pieces of onion over a leaf from a banana-plantain tree. That leaf with these described elements will help the patient when it is applied to the patient's feet.

The leaf must be tied to the patient's feet. Command the sick person to lie down (it is clear that because of the poultice being on the patient's feet, he must remain lying down).

The sick person will drink the decoction of chicory with lemon, as he would drink water, for a period of time.

This type of medicine must be performed every day and with a lot of faith until becoming radically healed.

Bless the plants, beg the elemental of each one of them to heal the sick person.

Heartburn

The troubling heartburn sickness can be cured by drinking vegetal teas of the following plants:

Chicory (*cichorium intybus l.*), dill (*anethum graveolens l.*), chamomile, gentian (*gentiana lutea*), centaury (*centaurium umbellatum gilib.*), celery (*apium graveolens l.*), dandelion (*taraxacum officinale weber*), wormwood (*artemisia absinthium l.*).

Any of these plants is marvelous against heartburn.

Simply boil it and drink it as an ordinary beverage.

It is advisable for those who suffer from heartburn to have more order in their meals. Therefore, such sick people must avoid flour, starches, and sweets.

They must eat only three meals daily and should not be gluttonous.

Heartburn

FORMULA:
Magnesia calcite   12 grams
Sub-nitrate of bismuth   6 grams

Divide this mixture into six portions, held in six pieces of paper folded over (three grams in each one). Take three portions daily, one before each meal.

Hemorrhoids

Make a decoction of thirty grams of plantain (*plantago major l.*) and thirty grams of mallow (*malva sylvestris l.*) to which the same quantity of the following powders must be added: "piedralipe," ground "cacho" (horn) and frankincense. The infected parts must be dabbed with this mixture with a piece of cotton, until totally healed.

Hemorrhoids

The hemorrhoid sickness is extremely bothersome, although very easy to cure. It is enough to sit on the top of a piece of ice and the problem is resolved.

Thus, application of ice over the hemorrhoids is the clue in order to make them disappear.

Hemorrhoids

Use daily three grams of "copaiba" oil, lemon (twelve drops of lemon juice), and sugar. Make it into a pomade.

Hemorrhoids

To apply ice directly over the hemorrhoids is the best of the best. Moreover, apply poultices of leaves of elder over the hemorrhoids. The problem of the hemorrhoids will disappear with all of this.

Hemorrhoids with Flux of Blood

Take four frogs and submerge them into almond oil. Broil this with fire, stirring it until you consider that the frog's extract has entered into the oil. The sick person will dab his hemorrhoids with this ointment. The healing will be inevitable; it is guaranteed because of the results obtained in diverse cases.

Hernias; Marvelous Remedy to Cure Hernias

We have always said that the plant "suelda consuelda" (*tradescantia multiflora swz.*) is a very efficient plant in order to cure hernias.

One takes the root of this plant after having traced a magic circle around it.

The elemental of that plant must be commanded to close the hernia of the sick person, to radically heal it.

In case you bought the plant in the market, then you must place it over a table and you will bless it and command the vegetal elemental to cure the sick person, to close the hernia for him.

The root must be cleaned in a very delicate manner and without scraping it. Then, it must be crushed within a mortar, receptacle, millstone, or pot. To crush means to mash the root very well.

Then, warm it up a little bit and place it over a cloth or a piece of clean fabric and apply it in the form of a poultice over the hernia itself. Change it twice a day.

Another Remedy for Hernias

The egg yolk is marvelous.

The yolk needs to be beaten very well, then add to it powders of watercress (*nasturtium officinale l.*).

Obviously, the plant called watercress is excellent.

One needs to make a poultice or cataplasm (of a very good consistency) with both the yolk and the powdered watercress plant.

Then, very patiently extend it over leather or a piece of very well cured and soft leather and apply it over the hernia.

That poultice must remain over the hernia until the poultice falls off.

During this time, it is advisable for the sick person to drink the watercress powder mixed with a good wine.

The elemental of the watercress plant must be commanded to heal the sick person, to close the hernia for him.

Hiccups

Hiccups are cured with sugar. It is enough to swallow a spoonful of fine grains of sugar very slowly and you can say goodbye to the hiccups.

Hoarseness

The decoction of pennyroyal stops hoarseness.

Impotence

Some people who have performed sexual intercourse in water have contracted sexual impotence, and often, paralysis to the legs.

There is another type of impotence that is known by the sorcerers and witches by the name of "nudo de la agujeta." This consists of a spell placed upon a man by a woman in order for the man to be impotent when trying to enter a woman.

These types of impotence are cured with the following formula:

Branches of "cuartillo," spearmint, "albahaquita," pennyroyal, and arnica.

Put these plants to macerate within a bottle of rum, which has to be mixed with the following combination:

Tincture of valerian	1 ounce
Cinnamon in powder	1 ounce
Camphor	10 centigrams

Bury the bottle for three days in a place where the sun will heat it up for the whole day. Thus, in this way the plants will disperse their healing essence within the rum.

The sexual organs of the sick person must be rubbed and humidified with this remedy until achieving a complete cure. The usual ritual before harvesting the plants must not be forgotten.

Impotence, Second Formula

Within milk, boil the fourth part of a goat testicle. In order to consume the decoction, add honey (bee-honey) to sweeten it. This serves for ten or twelve days. When your potency is recuperated, then study the books of Gnostic wisdom in order to learn how to transmute your sexual energy.

Impotence

The "cuaotillo" or "cuartillo" (*peperomia sp.*) with rum helps impotence. Place this mixture under the sun and consume it. Also the "viril de carey," which is a sea turtle, helps. It serves for getting an erection.

Impotence and Spermatorrhea

Go to a place where the plant that in Colombia is denominated "cuartillo" (*peperomia scandens*) can be found. Bless it and command the elemental to cure the sick person. Afterwards, collect the plant, a quantity equivalent to one pound (this must be performed while the moon is waning). Put it to macerate within one liter of firewater or rum. Then, kill two roosters and extract their testicles from them, which you must split in a cross on their most wide area. Then, add them to the

bottle of firewater or rum, which is already mixed with the "cuartillo." The bottle filled with all of this must be buried, taking caution to leave the lid of the bottle facing towards the east. Leave it for the space of fifteen days in maceration. Then, at the end of the fifteenth day, take the bottle out and consume three spoonfuls daily; the first dose is taken in the morning on an empty stomach. The affected person must nourish himself as best as possible.

Against Sexual Impotence

When sexual impotence is due to a simple sexual weakness, then it can be cured with male goat testicles.

PROCEDURE: Place these testicles to boil within milk. The milk is sweetened with sugar. Consume this milk as an ordinary beverage for ninety days.

The impotent patient will be cured; he will acquire a great sexual potency.

Impotence, Cerebral Weakness, Anemia

Macerate for twenty days, twenty free range (organic) eggs in lemon juice. Afterwards, add to them the following (ground) items:

Aromatic clove	2 ounces
Aromatic pepper	2 ounces
Star anise	2 ounces
Cinnamon	2 ounces
2 Nutmeg seeds	2 ounces
A bottle of brandy	

After fifteen days, add half a pound of beef lungs, which must have been previously dried under the sun and cured with salt. Finally, add half a bottle of white wine.

Inflammation

The nettle plant (*urtica dioica l.*) is a marvelous, efficient remedy against inflammations; it never fails. The inflammation of legs and arms disappears with the nettle plant.

It is enough to take some fresh nettle plants and to whip the inflamed area or areas with them for a few minutes. Afterwards, cover the area with hot baize or a hot cloth. Utilizing this remedy every two hours will heal the patient

Inflammation of Kidneys, Urinary Tract and Bladder, Rheumatic Illness, Lumbago Arteriosclerosis, Heart Disorders

The plant called spanish broom (*genista scoparia, hiniesta, ginesti, spartium junceum l.*), cures these tormenting illnesses as a matter of fact.

The flowers and leaves of spanish broom—the flowers preferably—must be boiled very well and the decoction must be drunk as an ordinary beverage until becoming healed.

Influenza

The teas from elder are magnificent against the flu.

Also, teas from the leaves and flowers of violets can be prepared.

Magnificent are the teas of guaiacum (*guaiacum officinale*), "pie de gato," slipperwort (*calceolaria herbeo-hybrida*), borage, eucalyptus, "gelsemio," lemon, "ambay," "anacahuita," etc.

These teas must be drunk very hot before going to sleep. Then, the patient will go to bed very well covered and will sleep peacefully.

Influenza, Grippe

Take Tetracycline M. K. in order to rapidly stop the influenza. This ends the rebel cough. "Masiquia," which is a flower sold in marketplaces, also helps.

Influenza, Grippe, Another Recipe

Take syrup of guaiacum (*guaiacum officinale l.*), suck the tablets of coal tar with "tolu" (*bombacopsis quinata jacq.*), perform injections of guaiacum oil of ten cubic centimeters.

Influenza, Grippe

Enemas with the decoction of the plant called horsetail (*equisetum arvense l.*) or "limpiaplata" (*equisetum giganteum l.*). Perform six enemas lying down on the right side and then on the left; that is to say, three on your right side and three over your left side. The patient will previously take a sitz bath with hot water. The duration of this bath can be ten to thirty minutes, according to the patient's tolerance level. Lie down enveloped within a towel. Then, when you get up, pass a wet cloth with cold water over the whole body and return to bed again until the body recuperates its normal temperature.

Insomnia

Those who suffer from insomnia must take wine mixed with seeds of the poppy plant, or make tablets of dried cilantro (*coriandrum sativum*) with sugar and eat them at bedtime. If there is no wine at hand, just the decoction of the seeds of the poppy plant is enough in order to give good results.

Intestinal Catarrh

"Calaguala" (*polypodium glaucophyllum kze.*), maidenhair fern (*adiantum capillus-veneris l.*), eucalyptus, wormwood (*artemisia absinthium l.*) and plantain (*plantago major l.*): drink this decoction four times a day (one dose).

Intestines; Against the Bowel's Flux or Intestinal Hemorrhage

First of all, it becomes indispensable to drink (on an empty stomach) for three days in a row, four ounces of the juice of the herb, which is very well known by the name of plantain (*plantago major l.*). Each time that this remedy is consumed, the following magical prayer must be prayed without any doubt and with a lot of faith,:

PRAYER

Tetragrammaton, Tetragrammaton, Tetragrammaton, I. A. O., I. A O., I. A. O.

With the 'OM' I enter into the garden of the Mount of Olives, where the Lord instructed his disciples in secrecy.

I find 'Isabel', who talks to me about the flux of her bowels. 'Isabel,' 'Tetragrammaton' I ask unto thee, I beg unto thee healing for my bowels.

I know that 'Isabel' wants the Pater three times and three times the Ave, Amen, Ra, Amen, Ra, Amen, Ra.

INDICATION: Once the recitation of the magical prayer is finished as well as the drinking of the decoction of plantain, then very slowly pray the "Pater Noster," which is "The Lord's Prayer," meditating upon the meaning of each phrase, of each word.

Now, after "The Lord's Prayer," do the same with the "Ave Maria," which is "Hail, Mary," by profoundly praying it.

Have faith in "Isabel" and you will be healed.

Love the intimate Christ and your Divine Mother Marah, Isis, Cybele.

Never perform any evil, love your worst enemies, and return good for evil. This is how you will live a healthy life.

Intestinal Formula

Gualanday (*jacaranda caucana pittier*) and the underground part of the stock of cashew tree: boil and drink these.

Intestinal Worms

Each morning, for nine days, consume the pressed juice of wormseed (*chenopodium ambrosioides*).

Intestinal Worms and Parasites

In milk, boil the leaves of "jayo" (coca in the interior of Colombia, *Erythroxylon coca*) and give the child a mug to drink on an empty stomach in the morning. The next day the child will take a purgative of castor oil. Thus, he will eject the intestinal parasites.

Jaundice

The sick person must inhale the vapors and also must be enveloped within the vapors of vinegar, which has to be cooked with maidenhair fern (*adiantum capillus-veneris l.*), oregano (*origanum vulgare*), sage (*salvia officinalis*), and pennyroyal (*hedeoma pulegioides*). This remedy of osmosistherapy is extraordinary in order to cure jaundice. The sick person must also wash his face with the decoction of these plants and his healing will be effective.

Jaundice

This tormenting sickness is easy to cure with the following formula:

A bunch of strawberry leaves, a good quantity of licorice, a good quantity of raisins (of good quality): boil all of these very well within a pot of water.

This decoction must be very well drained. Give it to the sick person to drink as you would an ordinary beverage.

Kidneys

The kidneys can be cured with the teas of the following medicinal plants:

Horsetail, "alfilerillo," bearberry (*arctostaphylos uva-ursi [l.] spreng*), spanish broom (*spartium junceum l.*), bermuda or scutch grass, "encino" (blackthorn), "linaria," juniper, corn silk, pine, licorice, salsify (*tragopogon porrifolius l.*), cuckoo-pint (*arum maculatum*), etc.

Any of these plants are useful for the kidneys.

Kidneys

Lemon juice and artichoke: take the cut half of an artichoke, or a quarter part (if it is too big), and bring it to boil until the water becomes yellowish. Then, add lemon juice and drink it three times a day.

Kidneys, Another Recipe

Consume horsetail (*equisetum spp.*), sage, rosemary, pellitory-of-the-wall (*parietaria officinalis l.*) and place cataplasms of milk curds over the kidneys. Children who cannot drink these decoctions must have the milk curds placed over their kidneys. Wrap a cloth around the milk curds in order for them to stay in place. Change the milk curds every two hours.

Kidneys, Another Recipe

The cataplasm of "venadillo" also helps. The "venadillo" is a plant of median climate and is very weak. The cataplasm must be placed for the space of half an hour for children. If they are mature children, they can tolerate up to two hours. Afterwards, take it off.

Kidneys

"Pitamorreal," "albaquita de monte" (*ocimum micranthum willd.*).

Kidneys, Affected

Prepare a decoction of rosemary leaves, artichokes (the flower head of the artichoke) and corn silk or corn hair. Consume three times a day or drink it as you would fresh water. It must be alternated with drinking fresh water.

SECOND FORMULA: Horsetail (*equisetum arvense l.*), corn silk and rosemary, ten grams of each plant. This must be consumed alternating with another beverage, which contains the juice of half an artichoke (the flower head). This must be put to boil. Then, add the juice of three lemons and consume it alternating with the former formula. The whole of this is good for the kidneys until healing the sickness. Consume daily, as well the juice of tomato: those tomatoes that have the shape of the apple.

THIRD FORMULA: Crush four ounces of purple garlic and put it to macerate within a half bottle of rum. Then, bury the bottle where the sun must warm it during seven consecutive days and then consume it by spoonfuls, the quantity of ten drops before meals. If this is too much, then only ten drops daily. Avoid meat and consume very little salt.

Kidneys, Irritation

The decoction of "canafistula" (*cassia fistula l.*, drumstick tree) with fennel immediately ends irritation within the kidneys.

The pressed juice of "cardosanto" (*argemone mexicana l.*, poppy family) beaten with fresh eggs also produces the same results.

Kidneys, Sick

The pellitory-of-the-wall plant (*parietaria officinalis l.*) is a panacea for sick kidneys. The elemental of this plant is small in stature and of a brown colored skin. He has the power of prolonging life and curing demented people. He also normalizes the menstruation.

There is also a parasite genre of the pellitory plant. This genre is a parasite from a tree called "cojones de fraile." The healing properties belong to the former plant and not to this parasitic type.

FORMULA FOR A CATAPLASM
OR ADHESIVE PATCH:

"Entre chipes," "lirias" or fine wax from "Mosca boba"
"Entre chipe de quisula"
"Angelita"
Milk of "copey morado"
Balsam of tolu
Ammoniac salt

Mix the balsam of tolu with the rest of the ingredients. First, beat the balsam and add a little bit of water with kitchen salt to it. Afterwards, add the rest of the elements until everything remains unified. Then, extend the cataplasm over a piece of cloth and stick it together over the kidneys. The patch will come off by itself when the kidneys are healed.

Kidneys; For Sick Kidneys

The most rebel cases will be healed by consuming three doses daily of the decoction of equal parts of pellitory-of-the-wall (*parietaria officinalis l.*), horsetail (*equisetum arvense l.*), rosemary, and sage. The first dose is taken in the morning on an empty stomach and the other two before meals.

Horsetail is also effective for the sicknesses of the bladder. The plants must always be blessed and the elementals must be commanded to execute the healing.

Knee Injuries

The inflammation that these injuries produce, which place the patient in danger of having his leg amputated, disappear with the following formula:

Mix equal parts of pork lard, ammoniac salt, and rock salt. Apply it hot over the knee with the security that the inflammation will disappear.

Lactation, Deficient

When mothers do not have enough milk for the nourishment of their children, then the following lactogenic aid will give them good results:

Reduce to powder forty grams of cottonseeds, which must be placed into five hundred grams of alcohol for the space of twenty days. At the end of the twentieth day it will be ready to use. Consume fifteen drops after every meal.

Leprosy

If a person who is overheated or feverish takes a bath, or if he bathes himself while with the flu, he can expose himself to suffering a flu in his blood capillary vessels, and the result is leprosy.

The blood becomes purulent and the disastrous biological process commences. In vain, attempts have been made to stop it with the famous "chalmougra" or with the derivative from "sulfates" and other preparations.

Leprous people die everyday, and there is no one who can cure them. The famous Colombian scientist Dr. Lleras Acosta classified Hansen's bacillus into more than twenty species. Through his laboratory investigations, he longed to know the chemical composition, which should displace the bacillus of leprosy and cure the sickness. Yet, Dr. Lleras Acosta was mistaken. Leprosy will not disappear by achieving the chemical decomposition of Hansen's bacillus or by inventing the reme-

dy that can kill it. Not a single sickness can be cured if the cause that produces it does not disappear. Thus, since this sickness is not produced by a bacillary infection, it is erroneously combated with antiseptics and prophylactics.

Cure the blood's flu, then the leprosy will disappear as if by magic.

Obviously, we must affirm that Hansen's bacillus live within a favorable environment. Thus, the moment when this environment turns unfavorable for them, then they irremediably will die, and the problem of the leprosariums will be solved.

Let us see the formulas we offer to cure leprosy.

FIRST FORMULA

> Gualanday (*jacaranda caucana pittier*)
> Sarsaparilla (*smilax officinalis*)
> "Zarza de palito"
> Mastic (*pistacia lentiscus*)
> Maguey (*agave americana l.*)
> Wormwood (*artemisia absinthium*)
> Sage (*salvia officinalis*)

Behold here seven hot plants whose elementals live within the Tattva Tejas. Cook them together within a liter of water and drink a big glass of this liquid before each meal. The blood is depurated in this way, and the liver, kidneys, and the spleen are placed into their normal activity. Tattva Tejas will eliminate the flu from the blood, which is the cause of the leprosy.

The ethereal waves of the fire are the only ones that can cure the leper, and in order to achieve this we need to handle the igneous elementals from these plants of this first formula.

Elementotherapeutical Procedure

At sunrise, make the magic circle from right to left around the gualanday tree

(*Jacaranda caucana Pittier*) and pronounce the mantra of the elemental of this tree:

Tisando, Tisando, Tisando

As in other aforementioned cases, bless the plant and command the elemental to cure the leper. Once this is done, take some branches (leaves) from the tree, facing towards the east.

For this operation, the Gnostic medic must cover his head with a mantle. When pronouncing the mantra "**Tisando**" he will mentally command the elemental to enter the organism of the sick person in order to cure it.

The elemental of the Gualanday tree possesses great erotic powers; he dresses in a dark green colored tunic.

The procedure for the sarsaparilla and the "zarza de palito" is identical, with the only difference being there is no mantra to be pronounced.

An incision with a knife is made into the trunk of the mastic tree; as this incision disappears, the sick person will be healed. Its leaves are collected after having commanded its elemental for the desired healing. The circle and blessing are done in the same way as the ritual that is performed for the gualanday tree; however, no mantra is pronounced.

The maguey is a Jupiterean plant. It has the three following mantras that must be pronounced:

Libib, Lenoninas, Lenonon

The rest of the ritual is done in the usual way as we have already stated.

Wormwood is a Martian plant.

The sage is harvested at night. First bless it and then yank it by surprise from its very roots. The elemental of the sage plant has a pale yellow colored tunic.

The sick person must try to personally perform all of this (to gather the plants as well as to practice all the rites). If this is not possible, then at home, he will perform what he should have performed in the country field, although with an obvious disadvantage.

We give the following formula number two. A glass of it it should be drunk after every meal. The elementals of plants of this second formula live within the Tattva Apas. Therefore, they are cold.

Second Formula

> "Ortiga del buen pastor"
> "Bretonica"
> "Verdolaguita"
> Fuchsia
> "Venturosa"

Boil them in a liter of water.

Before harvesting each one of these plants, the indicated rite (which we have already mentioned) must be performed on them.

Because the first formula is hot, there is the need to consume the second formula in order to avoid the irritation of the organism with the blazing fire of the Tattva Tejas. The fire and the water create the dense forms and equilibrate the organic life.

These two formulae from our Gnostic elementotherapy will be consumed for the necessary amount of time. The leper of third degree will be healed in nine months. The leper of second degree will be healed in four or five months, and a leper of first degree in fifteen days.

After the leper is cured, he must enrich his blood and cleanse his intestines in order to expel the dead germs.

Use the following formula:

Fluid extract of boldo	1 ounce
Fluid extract of rhubarb	1 ounce

Fluid extract of cinchona	1 ounce
Tincture of aconite	half of an ounce
Sulfate of quinine	1 gram
Simple syrup	1 bottle

This preparation will be consumed in little cupfuls, one before each meal.

This hot formula must be equilibrated with another cold formula. Consume the second one after each meal. Behold, here is the second one:

Cream of tartar	1 ounce
"Vichi" salts	1 ounce
Citric acid	1 ounce
Water	1 bottle

This formula corrects the digestion and refreshes the organism.

One cup will be consumed after each meal.

This treatment that I advise for leprosy is as exact as the Pythagorean tablet. Never has it failed and never will it fail, because it is as ancient as the world. It has been known since the dawn of our Earth.

The wise Indians of the Sierra Nevada from Santa Marta, Colombia entrusted this secret to me. They have cured themselves from this terrible sickness through its application.

A strong flu in the blood produces leprosy. It is not produced because of insufficient nourishment, or alcoholism, or hypertrophy to the liver... It is a flu in the blood... and nothing more than a flu.

Against the Terrible Leprosy

Leprosy can be cured with the following formula. Within the juices of these three plants—endive (*cichorium endivia*), hop (*humulus lupulus l.*) and wormwood (*artemisia absinthium l.*)—patiently humidify a freshly baked loaf of bread.

Clearly, it is favorable to add to these three juices equal amounts of vinegar and sulphur, which must be previously fused together (mixed together).

Then, add the third part of the juice of eupatorium and "ruda caprina," also called *aristolochia rotunda* in Latin and commonly "hierba sarracema."

Also add to the formula the twelfth part of cedar bark, the sixth part of the seed of the same tree, the half of hellebore and scammony must also be added. Expose the whole of it to the fire until achieving the complete evaporation of the aqueous part of the mixture.

Obviously, you will dab all of this medication onto all the parts that have been gnawed by the repugnant leprosy. If in spite of all this, some of those horrible spots still persist, then continue to dab the following ointment onto the skin of the patient:

Ointment

Rattlesnake fat, equal parts of ram and bear fat, the fourth part of caper oil, raw sulphur, and the sixth part of hepatica.

Unquestionably, the total of this must be submitted to a frankincense fumigation, and all of this must be cooked and re-cooked until reaching coagulation.

Finally, add a very small quantity of wax, so that this preparation does not harden. Normally, yellow wax is what is used for these kinds of ointments.

The leprous person can be cured with this prodigious ointment, even if his condition is already very grave.

This ointment must be applied to the patient every two days, until the total disappearance of the horrifying ulcers is attained.

This remedy is for external application.

The plants that are used must be blessed in accordance with elementotherapy.

One has to ask the Divine Mother Kundalini to command the Elemental Advocate, so that the latter can put the elementals of the plants to work.

Faith is the foundation of thaumaturgy.

Liver, For the

FORMULA NUMBER ONE: Decoction of boldo (*peumus boldo*). The patient must drink three glasses daily before meals. The first glass must be taken on an empty stomach.

FORMULA NUMBER TWO: Consume approximately fifteen grams of wormwood (*artemisia absinthium*) and fifteen grams of maguey (*agave americana*; the pulpy leaf of it). For the marvelous effect of the latter plant, there is the need before cutting it to pronounce to it the three following words:

Libib Lenoninas Lenonon

Then, bless it and command the elemental of the plant to cure the sick person. Each and every one of the cases, as diverse as each might be, must be performed in the same way; that is, bless and command the elemental to cure.

The sicknesses of the liver (which all of us suffer from to a lesser or greater degree) are cured with the following simple, yet effective formula:

Tincture of boldo	2 ounces
Tincture of gentian	2 ounces
Mint essence	2 ounces
Sugared water	1 liter

Liver and Gastric Visceras

Wormwood (*artemisia absinthium l.*) and plantain (*plantago major l.*): each person must prepare the formula with the quantity that is in accordance with his needs. The "almistillo," or "caguanejo" in "el huila" (Colombia), serves for the liver and leprosy.

The seed of this plant serves against any type of snake.

Liver

The leaf of the passion fruit boiled in milk serves to heal it. The passion fruit is a very pleasant fruit that is sold at fruit markets.

Liver, Another Recipe

The preparation of nutmeg with rhubarb and samson wine: close the lid of the bottle of wine and put it under the sun for two days. Consume three little cupfuls daily.

Liver, Kidneys, and Spleen Sicknesses; The Following Formula is Suggested

Tincture of boldo (*peumus boldo*)	2 ounces
Tincture of gentian (*gentiana lutea*)	2 ounces
Mint essence	1 ounce
Boiled water	1 liter
Sugar	a sufficient quantity

Drink this great preparation in little cupfuls, one every hour, until becoming totally healed.

Liver, Sick

The sick liver can be cured with the following tea:

A bunch of boldo leaves (*peumus boldo*), another bunch of lemon verbena leaves, roots of the plant called "mil hombres" (*cissampelos pareira l.*), and leaves from "carqueja" and "cepa de caballo."

These plants must be boiled and the water must be drunk, three glasses daily, one before every meal.

It is clear that all of these plants must be boiled together and the elementals must be blessed, commanding them to heal the patient.

The Gnostic medics must never forget the works with the Elemental Advocate, because the latter is the one who must command the elementals of the plants to execute the healing.

The Elemental Advocate immediately obeys the Father, who is in secret. Therefore, we must pray to the Father so that the Elemental Advocate will work.

Lumbago

Daily glassfuls of the decoction of the root of sorrel (*rumex acetosa l.*) and sage (*salvia officinalis l.*) are enough in order to alleviate this annoying sickness.

Lungs; To Prevent and Cure Their Peculiar Sicknesses (Great Panacea)

Take a gourd or "totumo" (*crescentia cujete l.*), make an orifice or aperture and place it above the fire. At the end of a short time, withdraw it in order to extract the pulp, which has to be strained so its liquid, juice or honey remains purified. Subsequently, make a decoction within a different pot of "calaguala" (*polypodium glaucophylum kze.*), "canafistula" (*cassia fistula l.*, drumstick tree), "vira-vira," senna, borage, root of "anamu" (*petiveria alliacea*), root of aloe, root of maguey (*agave americana l.*), petals of fine rose. The whole of this must be reduced to a liter, which will be sweetened with burnt panela honey (burnt hard sugar cane).

Then, this mixture must be mixed with the honey-juice from the pulp of the gourd and submitted to the fire again until it boils and the foam dissipates. When this intermixture takes on a black-like color,

then add honey (bee honey) until it is adjusted. Thus, it is ready in order to be taken by the spoonfuls.

Lungs

The plantain plant (*plantago major l.*) and lungwort (*pulmonaria officinalis*) must be utilized for all types of bronchial sicknesses and of the lungs. Put to boil (very well) a good quantity of lungwort leaves, along with an equal quantity of plantain leaves.

Consume one large glassful every three hours. Drink this remedy until becoming healed.

Malaria

The vagabond theories of official medicine in relation to malaria clearly reveal an exploitative and charlatan goal. The theory that states that malaria is injected by the "Anopheles" mosquito and that this female mosquito deposits its larvae in the stagnant water puddles is nothing short of a ludicrous statement. All the preparations based on quinine and all the prophylactic systems against malaria have become up to this day and age a great failure because the "causa causorum" of malaria is nothing more than the disharmony of the functions of the liver and the lack of vitamins.

We have evidence numbering in the thousands related with the former statement. Whosoever endures the inconvenience of taking a small trip along Colombia's lower Magdalena by following the river's shore will become convinced of this truth on his own. All of the inhabitants of that river's shore are people afflicted with malaria, and if we observe their nourishment system, we will then find the cause of their sickness. Those poor people only nourish themselves with cassava and dark coffee. The cassava only provides them with starch and a minimum quantity of saccharose. The dark coffee that they excessively consume irritates their liver, and when this organ is severely affected, then colds and fevers of malaria explode. Therefore, the hepatic disposition and the lack of vitamins are the unique and exclusive cause of malaria fevers, which in vain are persistently combated with quinine preparations.

In order to combat the colds and fevers, the decoction of boldo (*peumus boldo*) leaves is sufficient. Consume a glassful each half hour. We advise consuming beef eyes, cereals such as beans, lentils, corn, spring vetch (tare), haba beans, etc.

 Boldo leaves cure the liver, make the bile flow, and excite the hepatic functions.

The rangers from Arauca and Casanare (South America) cure themselves of "colds and fevers" with dark coffee mixed with lemon and salt. This procedure is slower.

The Arhuaco "Mamas" cure this sickness with the following formulae: "cholagogue" in branch, "tisaca," "capitana arconcito."

Menopause; Woman's Critical Age

During women's critical age, there are frightful irregularities in their menstruation, as well as disorders in the ovaries. Naturally, these bring on many other disorders. Therefore, women who are in their critical age must drink teas of the following marvelous plants:

Barberry (*berberis vulgaris l.*), artemisia (*artemisia spp.*), viburnum (*viburnum spp.*), juniper and also horehound (*marrubium vulgare l.*). These teas will alleviate them. The teas must be cooked, preferably in clay pots.

Menopause; Woman's Irregularities in Her Critical Age

Consume flowers and seeds of "arisario." Cook them separately, in other words, the seeds and flowers must not be mixed. We warn that the seeds of "arisario" must be previously ground before cooking them.

Each preparation is separately bottled up and must be drunk as an ordinary beverage. Alternate remedies, one cupful every hour.

Menorrhagia, Incurable

In order for menorrhagia to rapidly disappear, it is enough to perform cleansings with the decoction of the cortex of the pomegranate. That cortex must be grated in order to reduce it to a fine powder. Then, submit it to decoction.

Menstrual Delays

The "ansa" or "palo de la cruz" (*b. grandiceps jacq.*) can be harvested for it. When the leaves or flowers are cut off from top to bottom, they propel menstruation. Yet, when they are cut off from the bottom to top, they suspend it.

Menstrual Delays, Another Formula

Virginia elixir: This can be obtained in the pharmacies, generally in Colombia, South America. The woman has to consume 1 or 2 teaspoons of virginia elixir. It has a flavor like alcohol. This remedy provokes menstruation. When menstruation is flowing, then suspend the medication.

Wormwood also serves for menstruation and to open up the appetite.

Menstruation; Remedy in Order to Provoke Menstruation

Roots of sorrel (*oxalis spp.*) and madder (*rubia spp.*), a little bit of each one, then add a good quantity of strawberry leaves to the roots.

These roots and leaves must be boiled for a long time so that they may release very well their medicinal elements.

While the pot is set upon the fire, bless the vegetal elementals and ask them for the healing.

The sick woman will consume a glass of this remedy every morning until her menstruation returns.

Menstruation, Excessive and Dangerous

Acquire a very big, fat hen. Remove the guts and feathers from it and then fill the cavity with plenty of cumin seeds. Afterwards, sew it up with thread, so that nothing will be lost. Finally, put the hen into a pot of water and boil it until the meat falls off from the bones.

The sick woman will consume this soup in the morning on an empty stomach and at night, for seven days. Thus, she will be healed.

Menstruation, Retained

When menstruation is withheld, then it is advisable that women consume the decoction of cypress. However, it must be in small quantities, because in great quantities it can provoke abortion.

If the woman is sure that she is not pregnant, then she can then drink the decoction of cypress tea in good quantities.

Abortion must always be avoided, because it is dangerous. Whosoever provokes abortion, whosoever makes women abort, is a dangerous criminal of a high degree.

Delayed Menstruation, Bad Digestion, Children's Overeating, Digestive Colic

Rue (*ruta graveolens l.*) is a formidable and extraordinary Martian plant that normalizes menstruation or women's abnormal and delayed periods. Moreover, it has the power of combating digestive colic, children's overindulgence in food, and bad digestion, etc.

Ten grams of the leaves of rue must be boiled in a liter of water, boil it very well. Drink three glassfuls daily, one before every meal.

Take this remedy every day, until healed.

Mal de Madre (Mother's Illness)

Apply crushed nettle leaves mixed with cinnamon or myrrh over the navel or the vagina in order to cure this illness.

Mal de Madre (Mother's Illness)

The crushed leaves of verbena applied with pink oil or with olive oil (in case you cannot find the first one) mixed with pig's fat makes the mother's illness disappear.

Mumps, Goiter, Scrofula

Take a hunting snake and pass it like a massage various times over the mumps, goiter or scrofula and these will be healed.

The goiter will disappear in a very short time. Perform this treatment daily.

Also, this sickness is cured by using a necklace from the bones of the spine of that serpent.

Nasal Hemorrhages

BORAX POWDER: Use this as a nasal tampon. Parsley in maceration can also be used in the same way. If there is ice available, apply it to the head and forehead.

Nausea and Dizziness

Nausea and dizziness can be cured by drinking the tea of the following plants:

Sage, rosemary, lemon verbena, peppermint, lemon balm, orange or lemon blossom, gentian, passionflower, etc.

Neuralgia

Practice the rites to the elementals of the plants sweet basil, "guandul" (*cajanus indicus*), "juan de la verdad" (*aegiphila martinicensis jacq.*) and "ganamu." Afterwards, put them in decoction and apply baths to the affected area.

Nervousness

Boil equal quantities of lemon balm, parsley, and lemon verbena, then add some drops of valerian and half of a gram of bromide in order to consume three times a day. The first dose is taken in the morning on an empty stomach and the other two before meals.

Nervous State

The following plants will help: lemon balm, "albaquilla" (small basil), sweet basil, sweet marjoram, lemon verbena, orange tree flowers, orange tree leaves, five drops of tincture of valerian. From these plants, utilize the ones that are at hand.

Nervous System, Neurasthenia, Insomnia, Depression, Etc.

There is a marvelous plant called passionflower (*passiflora incarnata*) that is good for any of these illnesses.

Boil thirty grams of the stalks, leaves, and flowers for every one liter of water. Drink five mugfuls daily until becoming healed.

Nocturnal Pollutions (Wet Dreams)

People who suffer from nocturnal pollutions or abundant overflowing of semen must daily rub their genital parts with hot of chamomile oil daily, and before going to sleep they must place over their genitalia a patch of cabbage leaves with oil.

This oil must also be applied over the shoulder blades and dorsal spine (spinal column).

Another remedy that has been tested with astonishing results and that has not to be undervalued is the "orchata" (beverage) prepared with the seeds of melons. This beverage is sweetened with sugar and must be drank at bedtime. The kidneys must also be rubbed with cooking oil.

Nymphomania or Uterine Furor

There is a plant known by the name of "manzanilla silvestre" (chamomile), which is the body of a solar elemental that is intimately related with the wisdom of the snake.

This elemental is small in stature, with a white and gracious face, expressive yellow eyes, very intelligent and powerful.

When clairvoyantly observing this elemental, we remember the "Sagra" Maria Pastora, the great priestess of the snake. This great master of the Mayan ray uses a green tunic and she always carries within a drum a snake, the same color as her clothes. All the great initiates of the snake use a green tunic. The snake has seven secrets. Our serpent Kundalini also has these seven secrets, which are the seven cosmic days of the manvantara.

The great snake curanderos used to send a serpent to their enemies in order to perform their vengeance. If the snake has the command to bite the heart or the aorta of the curanderos' enemy, then the snake will accomplish the command and the enemy will inevitably die. The instrument for this magical operation is the "majagua" or liquid of the shoot of the plantain banana tree. These things are unknown in the cities.

Let us conclude with this short digression and return to the elemental of the "mnzanilla silvestre."

After commanding the elemental to extinguish the internal furor of the nymphomaniac woman, it is an essential prerequisite to kiss and caress this plant lovingly and tenderly before yanking it by surprise.

Then, place the plant on a plate and expose it for two hours to the light of the Moon when it is situated in the east, and for another two hours when the moon is in the west.

The husband of the sick woman will carry this plant around with him for a few days or for a few hours, and while in the act of sexual intercourse, he will humidify the woman's vagina with the pressed juice of the "manzanilla silvestre."

In this simple way, the excessive sexual erotic fire will be extinguished.

This operation must be practiced two or three times, and for a truly effective and accelerated treatment, give the sick woman the decoction of the plant to drink.

Obesity

Obesity is horrible; however, it is curable. One can become slim by eliminating bread, flour, starch, and sweets from the diet.

Obese people must drink teas from the following plants: horehound (*marrubium vulgare l.*), wild celery, "yerba turca," pellitory-of-the-wall (*parietaria diffusa* or *p. officinalis*), "frangula," "pesuña de vaca," blackthorn, "fuco," grapefruit. All of these are magnificent plants that do not damage, but benefit the overweight people in becoming slim.

These teas must be cooked preferably in clay pots. Drink them as an ordinary beverage.

Pancreas

Consume boiled plantain (*plantago major l.*).

Parasites

The decoction of the plant called wormwood (*artemisia absinthium l.*), when it is drunk for several mornings on an empty stomach, can eject parasites from the stomach and even the tapeworm. In the case of this terrible tapeworm, consume the pressed juice of wormwood, two or three spoonfuls mixed with ground peppermint.

Parturient Women; Afterpains

For the after-pains of the parturient women, place over the womb a bag that contains hot corn; when it gets cold, it must be exchanged for another hot bag until healing is attained.

Parturient Women; Against Afterpain

In this next formula, the parturient woman will burn orange skins and then reduce them to a fine powder that will be mixed with dry wine. The sick woman will drink one cup every hour, until becoming totally healed.

Parturient Women; Craziness and Epilepsy Because of Coldness in the Ovaries

(See also Nervous Epilepsy)

The first thing the Gnostic medic needs to know is the cause of the epilepsy, because this sickness has different origins. Sometimes a woman's epileptic attacks are produced because of intestinal parasites. Other times, it is caused because of perturbations to the nervous system, and many times because of consequences of flu to the ovaries.

The symptoms are different. In the case when the epilepsy is produced because of a cold to the ovaries, then there is no gnash-ing of teeth or froth coming out of the mouth.

FORMULA: Place one piece of panela (hard sugar cane) within one liter of water and let it dissolve for a period of 18 to 24 hours. Then add the following to it:

Tincture of rhubarb	1 ounce
Tincture of boldo	1 ounce
Tincture of cinchona	1 ounce
Glauber salts	1 ounce
Epsom salts	1 ounce

DOSAGE: One spoonful every hour. It is also urgent to bathe the feet with the hot decoction of the following plants: "santa maria" (*bryophyllum pinnatum*), mammee (*silvester guanabano*), oregano, pennyroyal and lemon balm (*melissa officinalis*). Before harvesting these plants you must bless them and command their elementals to cure the sick woman.

Air in the ovaries or a cold in them can make the parturient woman crazy. The treatment for this case is exactly the same as we have already indicated. As well, sitz baths should be done with the same decoction, or vapors applied to the vagina with the decoction of leaves and orange peel.

Parturient Women, Excessive Discharge After Parturition

The plantain plant (*plantago major l.*) is magnificent against excessive discharge that can occur after giving birth.

FORMULA: Plantain water mixed with a good wine.

Three spoonfuls of plantain water and three spoonfuls of a good wine must be mixed togheter. Then, add to the preparation an egg yolk that has to be beaten patiently.

It is indispensable to put this preparation over the fire and boil it for three hours.

The patient will consume this remedy early in the morning for three days. The patient must sleep a lot, every time that she consumes this remedy.

Pharyngitis

Pharyngitis is cured with any of the following plants: "alfilerillo," cotton, "mercadela," "palo amarillo" (*cusparia trifoliata h. and b.*), etc.

These must be drunk as an ordinary beverage until achieving radical healing. What is important is to have faith in the plants.

Pregnant Women; Recipe in Order to Stop a Blood Hemorrhage

In these cases, the Gnostic medic will utilize the following for the patient: seeds of a plantain plant (*plantago major l.*), root of bistort (*polygonym bistorta l.*), purslane (*portulaca oleracea l.*), coriander (*coriandrum sativum*), and sugar.

Reduce all of this to a fine powder. This powder must be mixed within a warm egg (within the egg). Then, the inside of that egg must be sucked; it must be totally sipped.

This is how the patient will become healed.

Pregnant Women; Non-localized Aches

Commonly, these non-localized aches of the pregnant women are due to the influence of some rays of the Moon. The sick woman will drink the decoction of the following plants in order to be healed.

"Huevo de gato" (*tabernaemontana psychotriaefolia h.b.k.*) or "hoja de luna y sol," and "hierba mora" (*solanum nigrumamericanum*). Three glasses of this decoction can be drunk daily, one before each meal. The sick woman must perform on herself internal vaginal irrigations or internal vaginal baths with the decoction of "hoja de luna," annatto (*bixa orellana*) and "ceibote" (named "ceibon" in the interior of Colombia).

The plants must be blessed before using them, and their elementals must be commanded to heal the sick woman.

Prostate

The prostate can be cured with teas from the juniper tree, ash tree, cypress, corn, lizard's tail (*piper angustifolium*), "pichi" (*psidium guajava l.*), uva ursi, "filependola" (dropwort), cubeb.

All of these teas from these plants are marvelous.

Prostatitis (Sickness of the Prostate)

The remedy for this terrible sickness is the plant known in the state of Magdalena (Colombia) with the name of "solito."

Harvest the plant in the morning, in the known ritualistic way. Boil seven of its leaves and drink the remedy hot. It is also indispensable that the sick man apply cataplasms of this plant (prepared with ammonia and table salt) over his prostate. This healing will be verified in a short time.

Pulmonary Catarrh

Celery, watercress, mallow (*malva sylvestris l.*), fragrant pine, pansy (*viola tricolor l.*), sage: consume the decoction four times a day (one dose).

Rebel Cough

To the decoction of white pine, white "caracucho" (*impatines noli-tangere l.*), borage, eucalyptus, and licorice, mix one ounce of tincture of aconite, one ounce of tincture of "drosera" (*nephenthes drosera*), one ounce of balsam of tolu and one ounce of tincture of belladonna. This preparation is consumed by spoonfuls, one every hour.

Respiratory System

Drink pulverized skunk liver mixed in a cup of warm water. This is an effective sudorific remedy and serves for the spasms, afflictions of the chest, catarrhs, fevers, and other sicknesses of the pulmonary tracts.

It has been told to us that skunk meat serves in order to cure syphilis; one must eat it until becoming healed.

Respiratory System, Rebel Cough, Flu, Bronchitis

Garden sage, *salvia officinalis*, jerusalem sage, *pulmonaria officinalis*, lung herb, lungwort, cardiac herb, virgin's herb, etc.: these are the various names for the plant that cures sicknesses like bronchitis, rebel cough, flu, etc.

Prepare it and cook a good quantity of its leaves and sweeten it with honey (bee honey). Consume the tea very hot, one glassful every hour.

Rheumatism

"Fenibutasona M. K.," 200 milligrams, serves as a very fast treatment. This is a pharmaceutical medicine.

Rheumatism

ANOTHER RECIPE: maguey (*agave americana l.*) with wormwood (*artemisia absinthium l.*): make the decoction, then squeeze in half of a lemon and drink it three times a day.

Rheumatism, Another recipe

Seeds of the poppy plant crushed with honey (bee honey). Also, "Fenibutasona M. K.," 200 milligrams, can be taken together.

Against Rheumatism

Any type of rheumatism, as very grave as it might be, can be cured with the following formula:

Sulphur	25 grams
Cream of tartar	25 grams
Rhubarb	15 grams
Guaiacum gum or arabic gum (either of the two gums)	350 grams
Honey	450 grams

DOSAGE: It is necessary to consume a spoonful in the morning and a spoonful at night of this remedy.

Unquestionably, it is necessary to dissolve this remedy within a glass of white wine or hot water.

The amount of medicine within the glass must be consumed daily, continually, until becoming totally healed. This remedy is infallible.

Rheumatism

The most excellent anti-rheumatic tea is the following:

Leaves of "alfilerillo," root of "mil hombres" (*cissampelos pareira l.*), leaves of ash tree, dandelion root, "cepa de caballo."

Without measuring and without too many complications, just put a bunch of each plant to boil within water.

One can boil all of these within a good pot and one must drink of the tea every day, as an ordinary beverage, until becoming healed.

Have faith, bless the plants, and you will become healed.

Rheumatism

Drinking the teas of the following medicinal plants can cure rheumatism:

Danewort (*s. ebulus*), nettle (*urtica dioica l.*), "alfilerillo," calaguala (*polypodium glaucophylum kze.*), dandelion, wild celery, horsetail, juniper, "espina colorada," "fresno," restharrow, guaiacum (*guaiacum officinale*), "mil hombres" (*cissampelos pareira l.*), olive, spanish broom (*spartium junceum*), "arenaria," *rubia spp.*, willow, blackthorn, sweet goldenrod (*solidago odona ait.*), uva ursi.

Any of these plants serve in order to cure rheumatism. These teas are all powerful.

Rheumatism from a Cold Corpse

There are people who have kissed and hugged cadavers. This action brings rheumatism of the joints that is not removed with any remedy but by using the peppermint plant, which must be boiled in a quantity of water that fits in a small mug (the size used for drinking coffee). Thus, in that quantity of water, put the plant to boil. Then, it must be mixed with another quantity of warm water, and with that quantity bathe the affected area or wherever the pain is occurring. Do this for at least forty days and do not eat meat during this treatment.

Rheumatism, Lumbago, Nephritis, Urinary Calculi

The plant called restharrow is magnificent. Boil this plant very well and drink the water as an ordinary beverage, every day.

Ringworm, Mange, Tinea

The pressed juice of the leaves of peppermint is applied in order to cure ringworm, mange, and tinea and other cutaneous physical eruptions.

Cataplasms of peppermint leaves with the crumbs of the inner part of bread mixed with honey are placed over the inflamed tumors.

Roseola

Roseola disappears by giving the sick person little glassfuls of milk mixed with lemon balm to drink.

Sciatica

Fornication is the principal cause of sciatica. Therefore, whosoever suffers from this painful sickness has to abandon the ominous, repugnant, and vile vice of coitus, if he wishes to be healed. Moreover, the sick person must nourish himself with a good diet based on vegetables, cereals, and orchard produce. He will also rub his knees and hips with vinegar; he will use a rag soaked in vinegar for this. This rag must be previously be smudged (smoked) with rosemary.

The intense pain that sciatica produces is similar to the pain that gout produces, plus there is the grave consequence of becoming an invalid, because the person reaches the crippled state. Therefore, for these grave reasons, it is urgent that this medication is used in conjunction with chastity. Let the fornicators say whatever they want, but know that is the cause, and that is the effect.

Unutterable suffering has to be endured because of fornication; this is how the human being has become more and more isolated from Mother Nature.

In order to complete this treatment, the sick person must drink beverages of the decoction of guaiacum (*guaiacum officinale*) and sarsaparilla (*smilax officinalis*) three times a day, the first dose in the morning on an empty stomach and the rest before their meals.

Scrofula

This troubling sickness is characterized by the inflammation of the lymphatic ganglia, and it is the first unfortunate step towards the horrifying tuberculosis.

The plant called radish is very well known. Scrofula can be eliminated with this plant.

Radishes can be eaten in salads.

Also, radish syrups can be prepared, and this is very simple. The radish syrup is prepared by boiling one liter of water with sugar and an sufficient quantity of radishes. A little bit of sodium benzoate must be added so that it does not ferment, otherwise it has be put inside of the refrigerator.

DOSAGE: One spoonful every three hours.

Sinusitis or Sinuses

The cause of this sickness is when a person bathes himself while sick with catarrh or a head cold. It is characterized by pain and bad odor in the root of the nose. The doctors used to scrape the gristle (cartilaginous tissue that divides the nose's nostrils). This would often disfigure the face of the patient, without achieving the cure, and providing no more than temporay relief.

We, the Gnostics, cure this illness in the space of eight days with the decoction of arnica, "rema" (*gouania polygma urb.*) and sage plants.

In order to harvest these plants, one must proceed the same way as indicated for cancer. Then, the plants are boiled in a pot of water. The hot vapor must be inhaled for one hour daily. The sick person will bless the decoction and will ask the elementals for their healing intervention.

Combine these inhalations with head baths, one every day, with the decoction of the following plants:

Orange or lemon leaves, "rema" (*gouania polygma urb.*), pennyroyal, "santa maria" (*bryophyllum pinnatum*), arnica and mammee (*mammea americana l.*).

In order to collect these leaves, the ritual already indicated must be performed and one must imperiously ask the elementals to perform the healing. When the sick person cannot personally harvest the leaves, then he will perform the ceremony at home, since (we repeat) the ones that cure are not the plants but the elementals.

Snake Bite

Drink the decoction of the following plants:

"Capitana solabasta," "capitana generala," "capitana silvadora," "capitana pujadora," "capitana lengua de venado."

Bathe the affected area with the decoction of the same plants.

When the case is very grave and the bitten person is believed to be dead, then with your hand try to yank the hair from the crown of his head. If the hair comes off easily, then the bitten person is already a cadaver. Yet, if the hair does not come out, then he is alive and one must rapidly operate in the way already advised.

Snake Bite, Rattlesnake

Drink and bathe the affected area with the plant "gallito" (*aristolochia spp.*).

Snake Bite, for the Coral Snake's Bite

Consume a decoction of the plant aristolochia by the cupfuls. Do not forget the ritual.

Snake and Tick Bites

It has been completely demonstrated that tobacco works against snake and summer tick bites, etc.

Simply perform rubs with the tobacco on those areas of the body that are affected.

Such rubs make the ill gas (which takes over the head and affects the sight) disappear.

Sorcery to the Head

Drink the decoction of the plant called "vencedora," and also apply baths to the head. The person has to immunize himself by carrying the plant called "cinco en rama" in his wallet.

Sores at the Edge of the Mouth

"Micostalin" syrup.

Spells

Green oil (from the pharmacy), powders of artemisia: mix these together and then apply to the area where the spell is felt to be.

Spells Placed on Houses and Homes

Collect the heart and liver of a fish with scales (the shad fish in particular), to burn for a smoke fumigation. Put these to dry under the sun or upon a low fire. Then, pulverize them in order to burn them as any other smoke fumigation. This type of odorous smoke fumigation works against any type of spell.

Spells on the Skin

Collect (in the way already prescribed) nine leaves of the plant called "solito." Collect the leaves in sets of three, and apply them in the form of a cross over the damaged skin. You must be careful not to damage the stalk of the plant in order for the elemental to cure the sick person of the spell.

Spermatorrhea

Spermatorrhea is cured with the tea of the plant called damiana (*turnera diffusa*). That plant performs prodigies.

Spleen, Against Pain of the

FORMULA NUMBER ONE:
Mix the ashes of rue (*ruta graveolens l.*) with goat manure. Cook everything in wine, then apply it as a plaster of the spleen.

The sick person must also drink a decoction of mallow (*malva sylvestris l.*) with powdered rhubarb (*rheum spp.*) for his total healing.

Also effective are plasters made with the leaves of raw cabbage that have been previously sprinkled with vinegar. Another plaster that gives good results is the plaster made with radish peelings.

FORMULA NUMBER TWO:
The pressed juice of tobacco leaves mixed with equal parts of castor oil and white wax give satisfying results when this mixture is applied over the spleen.

Do not undervalue these remedies because of their simplicity ot because they are inexpensive. The author of this book has made various tests with them and has achieved good results in all cases.

Spots on the Face

The spots on the face totally disappear by consuming the following great depuration:

Prepare the decoction of flowers and roots of maguey (*agave americana l.*), with wormwood (*artemisia absinthium l.*) and "bejuco de cadena" (*bauhinia excisa hemsl.*), sweetened with honey (bee-honey). The sick person must consume three cupfuls daily.

Spots, Black

Prepare sour orange with rhubarb powder within sugared water. Eating meat does harm to the person with spots.

Spots, White

FOR RUBBING: Multifungin (a pharmaceutical cream), honey (bee honey), a little quantity of sulphur powder.

ANOTHER FORMULA: Perform injections of bismuth, consume sulphuric water, and use a cream made with sulphur.

Sterility

Women who are sterile can cure themselves with "Curi" meat. Reduce this meat to a powder and consume it mixed with a good cup of hot chocolate daily.

Sterility, Women's

There is a remedy to cure the sterility in women that has never failed. Within the forest of the state of Magdalena (Colombia), there is a very wild bee denominated "tisula" or "gungura." The honey from this bee is infallible for the healing of sterility.

Mix the honey of this bee with aloe socottorina (crystals of the aloe, one ounce) and consume one little cupful every hour.

Many sterile matrimonies could have the joy of having a child with this remedy.

Stomach

People who cannot keep anything in their stomach can take "Gastrobil," which is a pharmaceutical remedy.

Stomachaches

A strong stomachache is relieved with water and sand.

The water and the sand are mixed together and put to boil. Afterwards, strain it and drink the remedy. The stomachaches disappear instantaneously.

Against Excessive Sweating of the Armpits, Feet, and Hands

There is a marvelous remedy against this tormenting problem, which is the sweating of feet, hands, and armpits, etc.

Formula
Five parts of neftol and ten parts of glycerin.

It is urgent to apply this lotion twice a day, and powder oneself with common and current starch to which two percent of pulverized neftol can be added.

This marvelous remedy must be applied by powdering between the toes and fingers.

Syphilis

All of the treatments from the false apostles of medicine to combat "treponema pallidum" have failed. No one knows which has caused more deaths: syphilis or the neosalvarsan and its derivatives that are used in order to combat it.

Patented remedies are invented daily in order to cure syphilis, yet the result is always negative. The prophylactic systems have served for nothing, because this sickness continues propagating itself in the same measure that it is combated.

We give the following exact treatment in order to cure syphilis of third degree in the space of fifteen days:

"Sanalotodo" (called "mosquita" on the coast of Colombia, *baccharis spp.*), "bejuco de anis" (*securidaca diversifolia blake*), "gualanday" tree (*jacaranda caucana pittier*), "bretonica," "ortiga," "maguey" (*agave americana l.*) and "guasguin" (*microchete conymbosa h. b. k.*).

The decoction of these hot plants will be consumed for eight days, one glassful every hour.

"Bertolita," "verdolaguita" (*kallstroemia maxima torr. & gray*), "tripa de pollo," fuchsia, and "paraguay" (*scoparia dulcis l.*):

The decoction of these cold plants will be consumed in the same proportion, also for eight days, after having finished the former treatment.

The sick person will bathe his entire body during the eight to fifteen days with the decoction of the following plants:

Anise herb, "coralito," "matandrea" (*alpina occidentalis*), "guanabana cabezona" (mammee, *mammea americana l.*) and laurel.

It is indispensable to perform the ritual for the plants.

Any syphilitic individual will be healed in the space of two weeks with these formulae, no matter how grave he might be.

Tapeworms

There is a very simple formula to eject tapeworms.

Formula:
Prepare a pap (a mash) with one hundred grams of pumpkin seeds, very well crushed, with very pure honey (bee honey).

Unquestionably, this remedy must be consumed on an empty stomach. The pumpkin seeds have never failed against the tapeworms.

After three hours, the patient will consume a soupspoon of castor oil.

Teething Tiger

If the tusk-tooth of this animal is hung from the neck of a child, then it can look after him during his teething process so that he does not suffer any irregularity in his body.

Tetanus

Apply purple maguey (*mikania guaco humb. & bonpl.*) as a poultice and also drink the decoction of the same purple maguey.

Tetanus in the Navel of Newborns

The cause of this sickness is when the navel is wrongly cured after being cut and when it receives an influence from a ray of the moon.

The healing of this sickness is relatively easy.

Fry a big onion head frond in cooking oil. When it is already fried, then add camphor (in powder form) and apply poultices over the navel of the child. Yet, before applying the poultices, apply fomentations of hot and cold water to the child, which must be alternated every five minutes for the span of one hour.

Thus, the Tattvas Tejas and Apas—that is to say, the fire and the water—will establish the organic equilibrium and will heal the child.

This remedy is safer than a million anti-tetanus or penicillin ampoules from commercial propaganda.

Tetters and Sores

On an empty stomach in the morning, the person must place a little bit of common table salt in his mouth. Then, wait for the salt to dissolve and then spew it out into a glass. Mix a little bit of soot with it, stir it until it forms a homogeneous paste. This paste will be applied on top of the tetters and sores.

Throat Damages, Children

Three lemons, one gram of table salt, one spoonful of honey (bee honey) and ten drops of merthiolate. This remedy helps to reduce the swelling of the tonsils.

Tinea

Collect equal parts of ground soot, sulphur, and marrow (from the head of a cow). Then, when it is very well mixed together, apply it to the head or to the affected area. This is always a marvelous remedy.

Also, pulverized cat manure mixed with mustard (reduced to a powder) and vinegar is a good remedy. This preparation is an unguent.

Tinea of the Head

It has been proven that duck manure cures tinea of the head. Dry the manure under the sunlight, then pulverize it and mix it with vinegar. Afterwards, rub the tinea with this remedy. The sick person will be healed.

Tonsillitis

Oil with bee honey and common table salt is an unequaled remedy for the disappearance of tonsillitis. If ulceration arises in the throat, then one must gargle with alum dissolved in water. If there is inflammation, then the gargling must be done with the decoction of wheat.

Tonsillitis

Tonsillitis is cured by gargling with the decoction of elder flowers (*sambucus nigra l.* or *s. canadensis*) together with poultices or cataplasms of fried onions with camphor and salt. The onions must be fried in cooking oil.

Tonsillitis

Boil fresh rosemary leaves within white wine. Gargle with this three times a day. If this produces nausea, then honey (bee honey) must be added.

ANOTHER FORMULA: Grains and shells of annatto (*bixa orellana l.*) must be boiled in water; this must then be placed outside, under the dew of one whole night. Gargle with it for nine days.

ANOTHER FORMULA: Three seeds of the colombian "pita" (*agave boldinghiana trel.*) or "enquen" must be cut open in a cross within pure water. Then, pink honey (found in Colombia, Atlantic coast) or honey (bee honey) must be added, then gargled. If the tonsils are very afflicted, then a cataplasm of "la madre del caracol" must be placed on them. In order to remove the inflamma-

tion from the tonsils, cook three lemons. Afterwards, take the juice out of them and add a grain of coarse kitchen salt plus a spoon of honey (bee honey) and ten drops of merthiolate. Dab the tonsils with the finger wrapped in a piece of cotton, or if dabbing with the finger cannot be tolerated, this concoction can be drunk.

Tonsils

Gargle with balsam, and touch the tonsils with petroleum mixed with honey (bee honey).

Tonsils and Throat Aches

(To gargle and drink)
Boil green rosemary leaves within white wine and sweeten with honey (bee honey).

Toothaches, Molar Ache

Cook a piece of alum, then humidify a piece of cotton within this water, and afterwards apply it to the gums, changing the cotton constantly. This remedy makes the molar ache disappear.

Toothaches; Mantric Secrets in Order to Cure

The affected tooth of the patient must be observed and the patient must divert his sight towards another place. Then, pronounce the following mantras while you perform the sign of the cross with your head: "**Onos Agnes.**" This secret is effective, because the pain passes away almost in the very act.

Tuberculosis

Tuberculosis is cured in fifteen days with the following formula: liquid from the shoot of the banana-plantain plant, pressed watercress juice and "iodocaine." The "iodocaine" is made with the following ingredients:

Iodine	6 drops
Tincture of eucalyptus	a sufficient quantity
"Guacanol" (oil)	a sufficient quantity
"Guayacol" (oil)	a sufficient quantity
"Creso"	2 drops

All of this must be mixed together. The sick person will consume it by the spoonfuls, one every hour.

The sick person will eat the plant called purslane (*portulaca oleracea l.*) for nine days. Purslane in salads is effective for the healing of the liver. It is also employed in the same way against sicknesses of the womb.

Tumors, For Many Types

Take a pilgrim-bottle calabash (*lagenaria vulgaris serg., cucurbita siceraria mol.*), which is a liana plant. Open it and fill it with rum. Then, close it with a cork and bury it underground for fifteen days. Ask Mother Nature to cook that calabash with the fire of the earth. Then, rub the affected area where the tumor is found and drink a spoonful of it. If you cannot tolerate drinking it as such, then dissolve it within water and drink it. (Two of these calabash can be buried).

Tumors (Formula to Eject Them)

Bitter "calabacito" with rum: make a hole in the "calabacito" and pour the rum into it. After fifteen days of maceration, give this remedy to the patient to consume by little cupfuls, one every hour.

The tumor will be ejected without the necessity of surgical operations, without exposing the patient to die in the hands of the surgeons.

Typhus

Typhus characterizes itself with having high and constant fever and an unquenchable thirst. Frequently, it is confused with an acute attack of malaria. Every hour, give the sick person to drink (as an ordinary beverage), one glass of the following decoction:

Arnica in branch, "cholagogue" in branch, sweet marjoram, wormwood, sage and "contra gavilana." Previously, you must perform the usual ritual.

Then, in alternation with the former formula, consume one spoonful each hour of the following formula:

Green onion	8 onion heads
Linden in branch	26 grams
Camphor	2 blocks
Water	1 liter

Cook all of this. Grind the camphor and add it later, when the decoction is already cold.

The fever is fought with antipyrine, one gram every two hours or six grams during the day. This is according to the physical state of the sick person.

Apply intestinal baths (enemas) twice a day made of water boiled with mallow and castor oil, or with the decoction of cañaigre (*rumex hymenosepalus torr.*).

It is also necessary to apply onion poultices on the soles of the feet in order for the germs of the sickness to leave (the onion possesses a great radioactive power). The sick person will be cured in the space of three to eight days with this complete treatment.

ANOTHER FORMULA FOR TYPHUS:

Antipyrine	10 centigrams
Acetate of quinine	10 centigrams
Chloral-hydrate of quinine	10 centigrams
Caffeine	10 centigrams
Tincture of aconite	20 drops
Tincture of nux vomica	20 drops

Mix these ingredients within a large glass of water and consume one spoonful every hour.

Remedy for Typhus

To quickly cure typhus is relatively easy.

Collect half a dozen very well salted sardine heads. Then, place them within a pot and mash them up as best as possible.

Afterwards, take a good quantity of the plant called rue (*ruta graveolens*). This plant must be previously blessed; the elemental of this plant must be commanded to immediately act upon the body of the patient.

Fennel must also be collected, and bread yeast as well. The fennel plant must also be blessed and its elemental must be commanded to work in order to heal the sick person.

The rue, fennel, bread yeast, etc., (mixed very well together), must be mashed within the pot. This must be mashed (with a great deal of patience) until it becomes a paste, which must undoubtedly be divided into two parts.

Certainly, each one of these two parts must be placed over a piece of cloth as a poultice, in order to place it on the two feet of the patient.

It is beneficial to remember that this marvelous compound must be previously sprinkled with hot vinegar before its application.

This is a prodigious remedy. The sick person will rapidly heal with this magical formula.

Ulcers, Cancerous

Wash the ulcers with the decoction of the fruits and leaves of guava (fruit of the guamo tree).

Ulcers of the Stomach

The effective treatment for ulcers of the stomach consists of consuming the pressed juice of the common plantain (plantago major l.) with lemon juice every hour. The dosage will be a five-ounce cup.

Ulcers; Gastric, Hepatic or Duodenum

Consume licorice; wet it and mash it. Do not eat red or white meat, or eggs. Nourish yourself only with milk, cereals, fruits, and eat meals without salt until the illness is gone.

Urine Decomposition or Putrefaction

The pressed juice of purslane (*portulaca oleracea l.*) abundantly consumed every morning on an empty stomach and cataplasms of the same plant, applied over the abdomen, cure that terrible sickness. The person must abstain from performing sexual intercourse.

Urine Retention

Boil within a liter of water half a pound of senna leaves, to be sweetened with honey (bee honey) in order to drink it as hot as possible. If the requested action is not attained, not to mention its efficiency, then there is the need to apply a catheter.

Urine Retention

In order to avoid the catheter, which is something that is not always possible because of the lack of methods or because of unforeseen or invincible inconveniences, then collect two ounces of horse manure. Dissolve it within a good wine, which has to be warm. Strain it and give it to the sick person to drink.

This procedure has cured very grave cases of urine retention.

Formula Against the Retention of Urine

Nuts are marvelous against the horrible illness of urine retention. Take a good quantity of the gristles or little walls (that divide the inside of the nutshell) and reduce it to a powder.

After reducing all of this to a powder, pass it through a silk sieve, a silk strainer or through a very fine fabric, with the goal of creating a very fine powder.

DOSAGE: During the last three days of the waning moon, one must consume one spoonful this powder. However, the powder must previously be left to soak (from the evening before, up until the dawn) inside the bottom of a glass, which is filled to the top with white wine.

One needs to drink all of this wine and powder very early in the morning on an empty stomach. Two hours later the patient will give himself the luxury of consuming a good vegetable soup.

This remedy must be used many times in the year, any time that it is necessary. The principal clue of this remedy abides in the rays of the moon.

The waning of the moon (in its last three days) has a formidable descending power, which can be used in order to combat this horrible sickness of urine retention.

Irritation When Urinating

The beverage of the decoction of mallow (*malva sylvestris l.*) With "canafistula" (*cassia grandis l.*) Efficaciously and rapidly cures this sickness. A beverage made from barley also yields the same results.

Lack of Sensation When Urinating

Burn bull or goat manure (it must not be a female goat or a cow). Then, mix the ashes with wine (of the best quality). The sick person will drink of this preparation until becoming totally cured.

Urticaria

Collect equal parts of the root of lemon balm, nettle, and sage. Cook them without sugar or any other type of sweetener and consume three dosages daily.

Uterine or Vaginal Hemorrhage

Prepare a syrup with wax, moss and leaves of "carey." Boil them together and drink in spoonfuls, one every hour.

Uterine Hemorrhage (in Serious Cases)

If in spite of all efforts the cessation of the uterine hemorrhage is not achieved, then do the following:

Provide yourself with three fragments of freshly excreted donkey manure from a farm. Then, within a rag, envelop the manure and place it to boil within a pot of water. Stir it well so that the manure dissolves. Strain it and give it to the sick woman to drink, a cupful every five minutes, until the hemorrhage stops.

Varicose Veins

Using external baths over the affected area, with the decoction of eucalyptus and walnut tree leaves, are known to be effective.

Varicose Veins

A clay cataplasm can be used. Rub the affected area and envelop it with a rag in order to hold it. Also consume boiled "suelda consuelda" (*tradescantia multiflora swz.*).

The "suelda" is a parasitical plant called "pajarito" (little bird). It yields green nuggets that become red when ripe.

Varicose Veins

Varicose veins are cured with horse chestnut (*aesculus hippocastanum l.*), "hammamelis," danewort (*s. ebulus*). These plants are all-powerful.

Warts

Apply the oil of the cashew or the milk of the fig plant over the warts

Recipe Against Warts

With great diligence, dissolve bicarbonate soda within a glass of water, as much as can be dissolved.

Then, in the morning at sunrise and in the afternoon at sunset humidify the warts with this marvelous water for two minutes.

Each time that the warts are being humidified, the following magical prayer will be recited with great faith:

> *Ae Gae, little wart you must go away, since the sun takes you away, OM, OM, OM.*

This magical remedy must be repeated for three days.

Wasp Sting

Camphorated oil is what has to be applied upon the affected area.

Note:

Within all that is evil, there is something good. Thus, some pharmaceutical preparations that have proven results can be employed.

We, the Gnostics, use the best of chemistry, as our Guru Huiracocha, professor from the University of Berlin, taught us. We extract from chemistry only what is essential, just as we harvest only the extract of reasoning, which is discernment.

The laboratories of the future will use the vegetable arcana and the most precious synthetic chemistry. Nevertheless, the human being must be liberated from that false materialistic science of this twentieth century.

Recipe for General Weakness

Place three fledgling pigeons in a pot to boil until the extract (stock) is taken out of them. Add one liter of curdled milk, and one glass of carrot juice, which is made by liquefying the carrots in a blender or by using a juice machine. Liquefy all of this in the blender and then strain it. Add a whole egg (with its shell) and liquefy it again. Add two little cupfuls of white wine and one little cupful of brandy and stir it by hand with a wooden mill (not within the blender). Take one little cupful daily on an empty stomach. If the person can endure to drink two little cupfuls, then let him do so. This remedy will end general weakness.

Weight; To Become Slim

Do you want to become slim? I advise you not to starve, but to become slim by eating very well. What is important is not to eat flour of any kind, no starches, nor anything that contains a sweetener...

Nourish yourself with vegetables and fruits. Consume beef bone soup so that your body does not become weak.

Horehound (*marrubium vulgare l.*), when consumed as a daily ordinary beverage, will help you to become slim. Keep yourself slim and you will see how well you will feel.

The fat, big bellied, paunchy, obese and massive bodies point to, show, indicate gluttony, etc.

Whooping Cough

Prepare of red pepper tea sweetened with honey (bee honey) and add some drops of tincture of lobelia. Consume one spoonful every hour.

A great sedative is "valim" for children. Another remedy is "florafenicol" or "pectp-sol."

Windy Colic, Abdominal

In order to cure a windy colic, it is enough to rub the painful area with saliva place a marinated tobacco leaf over the painful area.

Prior to this, it is necessary to moisten the tobacco leaf within firewater, tequila, wine or brandy, etc.

Women's Discharge

Use the decoction of the following three plants: "tatamaco," "cucubo" and sassafras (*sassafras albidum [nutt.] nees*) for washing or douching. In the case of virgins, this should be administrated by catheters. These plants invigorate and remove the inflammation.

ANOTHER FORMULA:

BORIC ACID ENEMA. Consume a purgative against parasites, such as (german) neo-biperbine; consume twelve capsules (this produces dizziness). Then, take a purgative of one ounce with glauber salts. Many discharges are produced by parasites and liver problems.

FOR OTHER DISCHARGES: Mallow (*malva sylvestris l.*), Borage (*borago officinalis l.*), Lemongrass (*cympopogon citratus*) with a spoonful of vinegar within a chamber pot. Afterwards, perform a cleansing with a jet of water.

Women; Bleeding Discharge and Leukorrhea

Eucalyptus with lemon.

Women; Leukorrhea or White Discharge

Vaginal baths with the decoction of myrtle and walnut tree leaves produce excellent results (with the condition that the previously indicated ceremony be performed). Do not forget, beloved reader, that if you yank the plants without this prerequisite, then the benefit that is acquired is very weak, since one is committing a grave error. Thus, the botanist becomes a simple vivisectionist of plants.

Women; General Aches

These are avoided when women stop bathing themselves while they are sick. Many of their non-localized aches come from that general bad habit of showering or bathing themselves when they are with their menstruation. Do not eat acidic fruits and do not eat meat one week before menstruation. Meat gives women a very bad smell. Women can cleanse themselves with warm water (cleansing their private part). Use deodorants, any natural intimate deodorant, etc.

Women; Any Type of Flux

Mallow (*malva sylvestris l.*), borage (*borago officinalis l.*), lemongrass (*cymbopogon citratus*, this plant is a herb that tastes like lemon), with a spoonful of vinegar of "castilla," vinegar or "guineo" vinegar. Boil all of this together for eight minutes and receive the

steam in a chamber pot. Afterwards, perform a vaginal bath with "fuente de gereben," which is a pharmaceutical medicine. Thus, everything will be okay.

Women; Disinfectant

The following plants can be found in the state of Tolima (Colombia). "Tatamaco," "cucubo" or "cubillo," and sassafras (this is a plant from which they take the "canime," which is a remedy for newborn children). Place these plants to boil and wash up with the decoction. This will take away any type of flux in general. A small spoonful of permanganate can be added to this cleansing.

Women; For Ovarian Aches

A beet and an onion should be crushed with a hand mill or in the electric blender. Take the pressed juice three times a day. The person who is allergic to onions can add lemon juice.

Woman; Sexual Frigidity

There are women who feel anxiety regarding sexual intercourse. Moreover, when this intimate relation commences, they feel repugnance for their male partner.

Certainly, it is a pathological, dissociating, quarrelsome, and unbearable state, which leads towards the destruction of affections and towards an inevitable divorce.

The Master Krumm-Heller (Huiracocha) wrote about this in his *Initiatic Novel of Occultism.*

The remedy for this sickness is the elemental of the plant called passionflower.

Contrary to that which occurs with nymphomania, the elemental of the passionflower (*passiflora incarnata l.*) has the power to light the erotic fire in those women who suffer from impotence or sexual frigidity.

The husband is the one who must execute the following. After having blessed the plant and commanded the elemental to light the erotic fire of his wife, the husband has to yank the plant from its very roots. Then, he will scrub the leaves between his hands and will embrace his wife's hands with his humid hands.

The embracing of hands will contribute to the major efficiency of this modus operandi.

This simple remedy will be enough in order to end the cause of many quarrels at home.

Women; Very Effective Formula Against Female Irregularities and Against Sterility

Bury (within a place that is heated by the sun for the whole day) a bottle, which contains equal parts of firewater and rum with the following plants: "contragavilina" (*neurolaena lobata r. br.*), "capitana," "malambo" (*c. malambo karst.*), dutchman's pipe (*aristolochia tomentosa sims*), "calaguala" (*polypodium glaucophylum kze.*), nutmeg and sulphur.

This preparation will be left under the ground for the space of fifteen days (no less). At the end of the fifteenth day, take the bottle out. Thus, it will be ready in order to give to the woman, one spoonful every hour.

It is good to note that before starting this treatment, the woman has to take a purgative of magnesium with "escorzonera" (*montanoa ovatifolia dc*). For that purgative you will proceed with the following formula:

Shred the "escorzonera," which is a vegetal similar to yucca. Then, you have to add magnesium dissolved in water. Thus, the purgative will be ready.

The sick woman must also consume three cupfuls daily of water that contains powdered orange skin. This powdered orange skin water has to be prepared in the same way as explained in earlier formulae.

Pomade Against Wrinkles

Two ounces of onion juice, two ounces of white honey (bee honey), one ounce of molten white wax: mix all of these elements together very well, then use it as a pomade. Apply it over the wrinkles.

Yeast Infection

The sick woman must constantly purge herself and perform vaginal cleansings with the decoction of myrtle, "moradita" (*caphea micrantha h.b.k.*, *caphea. racemosa l.f.*), and eucalyptus.

Yeast Infection

Yeast infections are troublesome discharges that produce suffering in many women.

It is necessarily urgent to burn a nutmeg seed very well and then divide it into two pieces.

Give the patient one half in the morning and the other half at night. This remedy is marvelous.

Healing from a Distance

The vegetal elementals can travel through space in order to cure sick people.

Magical Procedures

Place inside the magic circle the plant or plants that you are going to administer to the patient.

You must trace the circle on the ground with a piece of charcoal or chalk.

Then, you will concentrate on your inner God, asking him to give commands to your Elemental Advocate so that your Elemental Advocate will work with the vegetal elementals.

Afterwards, you will recite the Exorcisms of Fire, Air, Water, and Earth.

Exorcism of the Fire

Michael, King of the Sun and of the Lightning,

Samael, King of Volcanoes,

Anael, Prince of the Astral Light,

I beg ye to hear my call.

Amen.

Exorcism of the Air

Spiritus dei ferebatur super aquas, et inspiravit in faciem hominis, spiraculum vitae, sit Michael dux meus, et Sabtabiel servus meus, in luce et per lucem.

Fiat verbum halitus meus, et imperabo spiritibus aeris hujus, et refrenabo equos solis voluntate cordis mei, et cogitatione mentis meae et nutu oculi dextri.

Exorciso igitur te, creatura aeris per Pentagrammaton et in nomine Tetragrammaton, in quibus sunt voluntas firma et fides recta.

Amen, Sela, Fiat, Let it be.

Exorcism of the Water

Fiat firmamentum in medio aquarum et separet aquas ab aquis, quae superius sicut quae inferius, et quae inferius sicut quae superius ad perpetranda miracula rei unius.

Sol ejus pater est, luna mater et ventus hanc gestavit in utero suo, ascendit a terra ad coelum et rursus a chelo in terram descendit.

Exorciso te, creatura aquae, ut sis mihi speculum del vivi in operibus ejus, et fons vitae, et ablutio peccatorum, Amen.

Exorcism of the Earth

By the pole of lodestone that passes through the heart of the world, by the twelve stones of the holy city, by the seven metals that run inside the veins of the earth and in the name of GOB obey me, subterranean workers...

After concluding the four Exorcisms of Fire, Air, Water and Earth, you must pray to your Father, who is in secret, by saying:

My Father, my Lord, my God, I set myself towards thee, in the name of Adi-Buddha Tetragrammaton.

Lord of mine, by charity, by Christ, Agla, Agla, Agla, I beseech Thee, Ja, Ja, Ja, to command my Elemental Advocate and this vegetal elemental, so that they may place themselves inside the sick organ of (name the patient) in order to heal him. Amen Ra, Amen Ra, Amen Ra.

Afterwards, the Gnostic medic will concentrate on the sick organ and will imagine the elemental of the plant healing the sick person.

If the plants are many, then the vegetal elementals are also many. Therefore, the same magic work must be performed for each elemental.

Thus, this is how the sick person will be healed from a distance. The vegetal elementals can perform these healings from a distance.

Gnostic Medics

Gnostic medics are obligated to learn "White Nahualism" in order to visit their sick patients who are living very far away from them.

It is essential for Gnostic medics to travel consciously and positively with their physical bodies through the fourth dimension, each time that it is necessary.

The Gnostic medics who learn to travel through the fourth dimension will be properly assisted by the author of this book.

Therefore, we will grant them help each time that it is necessary. The Gnostic medics who delay in the learning of nahualism will be reprimanded.

We are not on earth to waste our time; we want wise medic-magicians.

We are tired of so many common pseudo-occultists and pseudo-esotericists that only know how to theorize.

We want concrete, clear, and definitive facts. We want medic-magicians who are capable of flying through the airs of mystery.

We want wise humans who really know how to handle the herbs and the elementals. We need medics like Hippocrates, Galenus, Paracelsus, who know how to cure with herbs and with elementals.

Each Gnostic medic must be a true theurgist, like Iamblicus.

Thus, only in this way, by having this type of Gnostic medic (who can materialize the angels in order to converse physically with them here and now) is how many people with unutterable sicknesses will be saved.

The angels will direct the Gnostic medics. They will teach them, they will provide them with the medicine for the sick people.

Conclusion

I have concluded this work of *Esoteric Medicine and Practical Magic.*

In the name of the truth, I affirm the following:

I am not searching for fame, honor, or money. What motivates me is simply the longing to humbly serve this poor, suffering humanity.

No one has the right to add or to take away from all of the formulae of this book.

No one is authorized to destroy this work.

I will now use the words from the "Apocalypse (Revelation) of Saint John" that state:

> For I testify unto every man that heareth the words of the prophecy of this book, If any man shall add unto these things, God shall add unto him the plagues that are written in this book:
>
> And if any man shall take away from the words of the book of this prophecy, God shall take away his part out of the book of life, and out of the holy city, and from the things which are written in this book.
> - Revelation: 22:18, 19

This is a sacred science, divine medicine, powers, sublime elementals, holy magic.

No one is authorized to adulterate, to add, or to take away from this sacred book.

Appendix

Prayers

Samael Aun Weor advises in some parts of this book to recite several ancient Gnostic prayers. He did not include them in Spanish editions of this book, because they are well known among Spanish-speaking people. However, he does list two of these prayers in his book *The Virgin of Carmel*. We, the translators, have included them at the end of this book to assist those who do not know these sacred prayers.

Hail, Mary

> *Hail, Mary, full of grace, the Lord is with thee. Blessed art thou amongst women, and blessed is the fruit of thy womb, Yeshua. Holy Mary, Mother of God, pray for us, who have the sinning 'I', now and at the hour of the death of our defects. Amen.*

Our Father (Pater Noster)

> *Our Father, Who art in heaven, hallowed be Thy name. Thy kingdom come. Thy will be done on earth, as it is in heaven. Give us this day our daily bread, and forgive us our trespasses, as we forgive those who trespass against us. And lead us not into temptation, but deliver us from evil. For thine is the kingdom, the power, and the glory forever. Amen.*

Apostles' Creed

> *I believe in God, the Father almighty, creator of heaven and earth, and in Jesus Christ, His only Son, Our Lord, who was conceived by the Holy Spirit, born of the Virgin Mary, suffered under Pontius Pilate, was crucified, died, and was buried. He descended into hell. The third day He rose again from the dead. He ascended into heaven, and sitteth at the right hand of God the Father almighty. From thence He shall come to judge the living and the dead. I believe in the Holy Spirit, the holy Gnostic Church, the Communion of Saints, the forgiveness of sins, the resurrection of the body, and life everlasting. Amen.*

Glossary

Absolute: Abstract space; that which is without attributes or limitations. The Absolute has three aspects: the Ain, the Ain Soph, and the Ain Soph Aur.

"The Absolute is the Being of all Beings. The Absolute is that which Is, which always has Been, and which always will Be. The Absolute is expressed as Absolute Abstract Movement and Repose. The Absolute is the cause of Spirit and of Matter, but It is neither Spirit nor Matter. The Absolute is beyond the mind; the mind cannot understand It. Therefore, we have to intuitively understand Its nature." - Samael Aun Weor, *Tarot and Kabbalah*

"In the Absolute we go beyond karma and the gods, beyond the law. The mind and the individual consciousness are only good for mortifying our lives. In the Absolute we do not have an individual mind or individual consciousness; there, we are the unconditioned, free and absolutely happy Being. The Absolute is life free in its movement, without conditions, limitless, without the mortifying fear of the law, life beyond spirit and matter, beyond karma and suffering, beyond thought, word and action, beyond silence and sound, beyond forms." - Samael Aun Weor, *The Major Mysteries*

Astral: This term is derived from "pertaining to or proceeding from the stars," but in the esoteric knowledge it refers to the emotional aspect of the fifth dimension, which in Hebrew is called Hod.

Astral Body: What is commonly called the Astral Body is not the true Astral Body, it is rather the Lunar Protoplasmatic Body, also known as the Kama Rupa (Sanskrit, "body of desires") or "dream body" (Tibetan rmi-lam-gyi lus). The true Astral Body is Solar (being superior to Lunar Nature) and must be created, as the Master Jesus indicated in the Gospel of John 3:5-6, "Except a man be born of water and of the Spirit, he cannot enter into the kingdom of God. That which is born of the flesh is flesh; and that which is born of the Spirit is spirit." The Solar Astral Body is created as a result of the Third Initiation of Major Mysteries

(Serpents of Fire), and is perfected in the Third Serpent of Light. In Tibetan Buddhism, the Solar Astral Body is known as the illusory body (sgyu-lus). This body is related to the emotional center and to the sephirah Hod.

"Really, only those who have worked with the Maithuna (White Tantra) for many years can possess the Astral Body." - Samael Aun Weor, *The Elimination of Satan's Tail*

Atman: (Sanskrit, literally "self") An ancient and important word that is grossly misinterpreted in much of Hinduism and Buddhism. Many have misunderstood this word as referring to a permanently existing self or soul. Yet the true meaning is otherwise.

"Brahman, Self, Purusha, Chaitanya, Consciousness, God, Atman, Immortality, Freedom, Perfection, Bliss, Bhuma or the unconditioned are synonymous terms." - Swami Sivananva

Thus, Atman as "self" refers to a state of being "unconditioned," which is related to the Absolute, the Ain Soph, or the Shunyata (Emptiness). Thus, Atman refers to the Innermost, the Spirit, the Son of God, who longs to return to that which is beyond words.

"Atman, in Himself, is the ineffable Being, the one who is beyond time and eternity, without end of days. He does not die, neither reincarnates (the ego is what returns), but Atman is absolutely perfect." - Samael Aun Weor

In general use, the term Atman can refer to the Spirit or sephirah Chesed.

"The Being Himself is Atman, the Ineffable. If we commit the error of giving the Being the qualifications of superior "I," alter ego, subliminal "I," or divine ego, etc., we commit blasphemy, because That which is Divine, the Reality, can never fall into the heresy of separability. Superior and inferior are two sections of the same thing. Superior "I" or inferior "I" are two sections of the same pluralized ego (Satan). The Being is the Being, and the reason for the Being to be is to be the same Being. The

Being transcends the personality, the "I," and individuality." Samael Aun Weor

"Bliss is the essential nature of man. The central fact of man's being is his inherent divinity. Man's essential nature is divine, the awareness of which he has lost because of his animal propensities and the veil of ignorance. Man, in his ignorance, identifies himself with the body, mind, Prana and the senses. Transcending these, he becomes one with Brahman or the Absolute who is pure bliss. Brahman or the Absolute is the fullest reality, the completest Consciousness. That beyond which there is nothing, that which is the innermost Self of all is Atman or Brahman. The Atman is the common Consciousness in all beings. A thief, a prostitute, a scavenger, a king, a rogue, a saint, a dog, a cat, a rat-all have the same common Atman. There is apparent, fictitious difference in bodies and minds only. There are differences in colours and opinions. But, the Atman is the same in all. If you are very rich, you can have a steamer, a train, an airship of your own for your own selfish interests. But, you cannot have an Atman of your own. The Atman is common to all. It is not an individual's sole registered property. The Atman is the one amidst the many. It is constant amidst the forms which come and go. It is the pure, absolute, essential Consciousness of all the conscious beings. The source of all life, the source of all knowledge is the Atman, thy innermost Self. This Atman or Supreme Soul is transcendent, inexpressible, uninferable, unthinkable, indescribable, the ever-peaceful, all-blissful. There is no difference between the Atman and bliss. The Atman is bliss itself. God, perfection, peace, immortality, bliss are one. The goal of life is to attain perfection, immortality or God. The nearer one approaches the Truth, the happier one becomes. For, the essential nature of Truth is positive, absolute bliss. There is no bliss in the finite. Bliss is only in the Infinite. Eternal bliss can be had only from the eternal Self. To know the Self is to enjoy eternal bliss and everlasting peace. Self-realisation bestows eternal existence, absolute knowledge, and perennial bliss. None can be saved without Self-realisation. The quest for the Absolute should be undertaken even sacrificing the

dearest object, even life, even courting all pain. Study philosophical books as much as you like, deliver lectures and lectures throughout your global tour, remain in a Himalayan cave for one hundred years, practise Pranayama for fifty years, you cannot attain emancipation without the realisation of the oneness of the Self." - Swami Sivananda

Buddhi: (Sanskrit, literally "intelligence") An aspect of mind.

"Buddhi is pure [superior] reason. The seat of Buddhi is just below the crown of the head in the Pineal Gland of the brain. Buddhi is manifested only in those persons who have developed right intuitive discrimination or Viveka. The ordinary reason of the worldly people is termed practical reason, which is dense and has limitations... Sankhya Buddhi or Buddhi in the light of Sankhya philosophy is will and intellect combined. Mind is microcosm. Mind is Maya. Mind occupies an intermediate state between Prakriti and Purusha, matter and Spirit." - Swami Sivananda, *Yoga in Daily Life*

"When the diverse, confining sheaths of the Atma have been dissolved by Sadhana, when the different Vrittis of the mind have been controlled by mental drill or gymnastic, when the conscious mind is not active, you enter the realm of spirit life, the super-conscious mind where Buddhi and pure reason and intuition, the faculty of direct cognition of Truth, manifest. You pass into the kingdom of peace where there is none to speak, you will hear the voice of God which is very clear and pure and has an upward tendency. Listen to the voice with attention and interest. It will guide you. It is the voice of God." - Swami Sivananda, *Essence of Yoga*

In Kabbalah: The feminine Spiritual Soul, related to the sephirah Geburah. Symbolized throughout world literature, notably as Helen of Troy, Beatrice in The Divine Comedy, and Beth-sheba (Hebrew, literally "daughter of seven") in the Old Testament. The Divine or Spiritual Soul is the feminine soul of the Innermost (Atman), or his "daughter." All the strength, all the power of the Gods and Goddesses resides in Buddhi / Geburah, Cosmic Consciousness, as within a glass of alabaster where the flame of the Inner Being (Gedulah, Atman the Ineffable) is always burning.

Chakra: (Sanskrit) Literally, "wheel." The chakras are subtle centers of energetic transformation. There are hundreds of chakras in our hidden physiology, but seven primary ones related to the awakening of consciousness.

"The Chakras are centres of Shakti as vital force... The Chakras are not perceptible to the gross senses. Even if they were perceptible in the living body which they help to organise, they disappear with the disintegration of organism at death." - Swami Sivananda, *Kundalini Yoga*

"The chakras are points of connection through which the divine energy circulates from one to another vehicle of the human being." - Samael Aun Weor, *Aztec Christic Magic*

Christ: Derived from the Greek Christos, "the Anointed One," and Krestos, whose esoteric meaning is "fire." The word Christ is a title, not a personal name.

"Indeed, Christ is a Sephirothic Crown (Kether, Chokmah and Binah) of incommensurable wisdom, whose purest atoms shine within Chokmah, the world of the Ophanim. Christ is not the Monad, Christ is not the Theosophical Septenary; Christ is not the Jivan-Atman. Christ is the Central Sun. Christ is the ray that unites us to the Absolute." - Samael Aun Weor, *Tarot and Kabbalah*

Consciousness: "Wherever there is life, there exists the consciousness. Consciousness is inherent to life as humidity is inherent to water." - Samael Aun Weor, *Fundamental Notions of Endocrinology and Criminology*

From various dictionaries: 1. The state of being conscious; knowledge of one's own existence, condition, sensations, mental operations, acts, etc. 2. Immediate knowledge or perception of the presence of any object, state, or sensation. 3. An alert cognitive state in which you are aware of yourself and your situation. In Universal Gnosticism, the range of potential consciousness is allegorized in the Ladder of Jacob, upon which the angels ascend and descend. Thus there are higher and lower levels of consciousness, from the level of demons at the bottom, to highly realized angels in the heights.

"It is vital to understand and develop the conviction that consciousness has the potential to increase to an infinite degree." - The 14th Dalai Lama.

"Light and consciousness are two phenomena of the same thing; to a lesser degree of consciousness, corresponds a lesser degree of light; to a greater degree of consciousness, a greater degree of light." - Samael Aun Weor, *The Esoteric Treatise of Hermetic Astrology*

Divine Mother: "Among the Aztecs, she was known as Tonantzin, among the Greeks as chaste Diana. In Egypt she was Isis, the Divine Mother, whose veil no mortal has lifted. There is no doubt at all that esoteric Christianity has never forsaken the worship of the Divine Mother Kundalini. Obviously she is Marah, or better said, RAM-IO, MARY. What orthodox religions did not specify, at least with regard to the exoteric or public circle, is the aspect of Isis in her individual human form. Clearly, it was taught only in secret to the Initiates that this Divine Mother exists individually within each human being. It cannot be emphasized enough that Mother-God, Rhea, Cybele, Adonia, or whatever we wish to call her, is a variant of our own individual Being in the here and now. Stated explicitly, each of us has our own particular, individual Divine Mother." - Samael Aun Weor, *The Great Rebellion*

"Devi Kundalini, the Consecrated Queen of Shiva, our personal Divine Cosmic Individual Mother, assumes five transcendental mystic aspects in every creature, which we must enumerate:

1. The unmanifested Prakriti

2. The chaste Diana, Isis, Tonantzin, Maria or better said Ram-Io

3. The terrible Hecate, Persephone, Coatlicue, queen of the infernos and death; terror of love and law

4. The special individual Mother Nature, creator and architect of our physical organism

5. The Elemental Enchantress to whom we owe every vital impulse, every instinct." - Samael Aun Weor, *The Mystery of the Golden Blossom*

Drukpa: (Also known variously as Druk-pa, Dug-pa, Brugpa, Dag dugpa or Dad dugpa) The term Drukpa comes from from Dzongkha and Tibetan 'brug yul, which means "country of Bhutan," and is composed of Druk, "dragon," and pa, "person." In Asia, the word refers to the people of Bhutan, a country between India and Tibet. Drukpa can also refer to a large sect of Buddhism which broke from the Kagyug-pa "the Ones of the Oral Tradition." They considered themselves as the heirs of the indian Gurus: their teaching, which goes back to Vajradhara, was conveyed through Dakini, from Naropa to Marpa and then to the ascetic and mystic poet Milarepa. Later on, Milarepa's disciples founded new monasteries, and new threads appeared, among which are the Karmapa and the Drukpa. All those schools form the Kagyug-pa order, in spite of episodic internal quarrels and extreme differences in practice. The Drukpa sect is recognized by their ceremonial large red hats, but it should be known that they are not the only "Red Hat" group (the Nyingmas, founded by Padmasambhava, also use red hats). The Drukpas have established a particular worship of the Dorje (Vajra, or thunderbolt, a symbol of the phallus). Samael Aun Weor wrote repeatedly in many books that the "Drukpas" practice and teach Black Tantra, by means of the expelling of the sexual energy. If we analyze the word, it is clear that he is referring to "Black Dragons," or people who practice Black Tantra. He was not referring to all the people of Bhutan, or all members of the Buddhist Drukpa sect. Such a broad condemnation would be as ridiculous as the one made by those who condemn all Jews for the crucifixion of Jesus.

Ego: The multiplicity of contradictory psychological elements that we have inside are in their sum the "ego." Each one is also called "an ego" or an "I." Every ego is a psychological defect which produces suffering. The ego is three (related to our Three Brains or three centers of psychological processing), seven (capital sins), and legion (in their infinite variations).

"The ego is the root of ignorance and pain." - Samael Aun Weor, *The Esoteric Treatise of Hermetic Astrology*

"The Being and the ego are incompatible. The Being and the ego are like water and oil. They can never be mixed... The annihilation of the psychic aggregates (egos) can be made possible only by radically comprehending our errors through meditation and by the evident Self-reflection of the Being." - Samael Aun Weor, *The Pistis Sophia Unveiled*

Fornication: Originally, the term fornication was derived from the Indo-European word gwher, whose meanings relate to heat and burning (the full explanation can be found online at http://sacred-sex.org/terminology/fornication). Fornication means to make the heat (solar fire) of the seed (sexual power) leave the body through voluntary orgasm. Any voluntary orgasm is fornication, whether between a married man and woman, or an unmarried man and woman, or through masturbation, or in any other case; this is explained by Moses: "A man from whom there is a discharge of semen, shall immerse all his flesh in water, and he shall remain unclean until evening. And any garment or any leather [object] which has semen on it, shall be immersed in water, and shall remain unclean until evening. A woman with whom a man cohabits, whereby there was [a discharge of] semen, they shall immerse in water, and they shall remain unclean until evening." - Leviticus 15:16-18

To fornicate is to spill the sexual energy through the orgasm. Those who "deny themselves" restrain the sexual energy, and "walk in the midst of the fire" without being burned. Those who restrain the sexual energy, who renounce the orgasm, remember God in themselves, and do not defile themselves with animal passion, "for the temple of God is holy, which temple ye are."

"Whosoever is born of God doth not commit sin; for his seed remaineth in him: and he cannot sin, because he is born of God." - 1 John 3:9

This is why neophytes always took a vow of sexual abstention, so that they could prepare themselves for marriage, in which they would have sexual relations but not release the sexual energy through the orgasm. This is why Paul advised:

"...they that have wives be as though they had none..." - I Corinthians 7:29

"A fornicator is an individual who has intensely accustomed his genital organs to copulate (with orgasm). Yet, if the same individual changes his custom of copulation to the custom of no copulation, then he transforms himself into a chaste person. We have as an example the astonishing case of Mary Magdalene, who was a famous prostitute. Mary Magdalene became the famous Saint Mary Magdalene, the repented prostitute. Mary Magdalene became the chaste disciple [and wife] of Christ." - Samael Aun Weor, *The Revolution of Beelzebub*

Gnosis: (Greek) Knowledge.

1. The word Gnosis refers to the knowledge we acquire through our own experience, as opposed to knowledge that we are told or believe in. Gnosis - by whatever name in history or culture - is conscious, experiential knowledge, not merely intellectual or conceptual knowledge, belief, or theory. This term is synonymous with the Hebrew "daath" and the Sanskrit "jna."

2. The tradition that embodies the core wisdom or knowledge of humanity.

"Gnosis is the flame from which all religions sprouted, because in its depth Gnosis is religion. The word "religion" comes from the Latin word "religare," which implies "to link the Soul to God"; so Gnosis is the very pure flame from where all religions sprout, because Gnosis is knowledge, Gnosis is wisdom." - Samael Aun Weor, *The Esoteric Path*

"The secret science of the Sufis and of the Whirling Dervishes is within Gnosis. The secret doctrine of Buddhism and of Taoism is within Gnosis. The sacred magic of the Nordics is within Gnosis. The wisdom of Hermes, Buddha, Confucius, Mohammed and Quetzalcoatl, etc., etc., is within Gnosis. Gnosis is the doctrine of Christ." - Samael Aun Weor, *The Revolution of Beelzebub*

Innermost: "Our real Being is of a universal nature. Our real Being is neither a kind of superior nor inferior "I." Our real Being is impersonal, universal, divine. He transcends every concept of "I," me, myself, ego, etc., etc." - Samael Aun Weor, *The Perfect Matrimony*

Also known as Atman, the Spirit, Chesed, our own individual interior divine Father.

"The Innermost is the ardent flame of Horeb. In accordance with Moses, the Innermost is the Ruach Elohim (the Spirit of God) who sowed the waters in the beginning of the world. He is the Sun King, our Divine Monad, the Alter-Ego of Cicerone." - Samael Aun Weor, *The Revolution of Beelzebub*

Internal Worlds: The many dimensions beyond the physical world. These dimensions are both subjective and objective. To know the objective internal worlds (the Astral Plane, or Nirvana, or the Klipoth) one must first know one's own personal, subjective internal worlds, because the two are intimately associated.

"Whosoever truly wants to know the internal worlds of the planet Earth or of the solar system or of the galaxy in which we live, must previously know his intimate world, his individual, internal life, his own internal worlds. Man, know thyself, and thou wilt know the Universe and its Gods. The more we explore this internal world called "myself," the more we will comprehend that we simultaneously live in two worlds, in two realities, in two confines: the external and the internal. In the same way that it is indispensable for one to learn how to walk in the external world so as not to fall down into a precipice, or not get lost in the streets of the city, or to select one's friends, or not associate with the perverse ones, or not eat poison, etc.; likewise, through the psychological work upon oneself we learn how to walk in the internal world, which is explorable only through Self-observation." - Samael Aun Weor, *Revolutionary Psychology*

Through the work in Self-observation, we develop the capacity to awaken where previously we were asleep: including in the objective internal worlds.

Kundalini: "Kundalini, the serpent power or mystic fire, is the primordial energy or Sakti that lies dormant or sleeping in the Muladhara Chakra, the centre of the body. It is called the serpentine or annular power on account of serpentine form. It is an electric fiery occult power, the great pristine force which underlies all organic and inorganic matter. Kundalini is the cosmic power in individual bodies. It is not a material force like electricity, magnetism, centripetal or centrifugal force. It is a spiritual potential Sakti or cosmic power. In reality it has no form. [...] O Divine Mother Kundalini, the Divine Cosmic Energy that is hidden in men! Thou art Kali, Durga, Adisakti, Rajarajeswari, Tripurasundari, Maha-Lakshmi, Maha-Sarasvati! Thou hast put on all these names and forms. Thou hast manifested as Prana, electricity, force, magnetism, cohesion, gravitation in this universe. This whole universe rests in Thy bosom. Crores of salutations unto thee. O Mother of this world! Lead me on to open the Sushumna Nadi and take Thee along the Chakras to Sahasrara Chakra and to merge myself in Thee and Thy consort, Lord Siva. Kundalini Yoga is that Yoga which treats of Kundalini Sakti, the six centres of spiritual energy (Shat Chakras), the arousing of the sleeping Kundalini Sakti and its union with Lord Siva in Sahasrara Chakra, at the crown of the head. This is an exact science. This is also known as Laya Yoga. The six centres are pierced (Chakra Bheda) by the passing of Kundalini Sakti to the top of the head. 'Kundala' means 'coiled'. Her form is like a coiled serpent. Hence the name Kundalini." - Swami Sivananda, *Kundalini Yoga*

"Kundalini is a compound word: Kunda reminds us of the abominable "Kundabuffer organ," and lini is an Atlantean term meaning termination. Kundalini means "the termination of the abominable Kundabuffer organ." In this case, it is imperative not to confuse Kundalini with Kundabuffer." - Samael Aun Weor, *The Great Rebellion*

These two forces, one positive and ascending, and one negative and descending, are symbolized in the Bible in the book of Numbers (the story of the Serpent of Brass). The Kundalini is "The power of life."- from the Theosophical Glossary. The sexual fire that is at the base of all life.

"The ascent of the Kundalini along the spinal cord is achieved very slowly in accordance with the merits of the heart. The fires of the heart control the miraculous development of the sacred serpent. Devi Kundalini is not something mechanical as many suppose; the igneous serpent is only awakened with genuine Love between husband and wife, and it will never rise up along the medullar canal of adulterers." -Samael Aun Weor, *The Mystery of the Golden Blossom*

"The decisive factor in the progress, development and evolution of the Kundalini is ethics." - Samael Aun Weor, *The Revolution of Beelzebub*

"Until not too long ago, the majority of spiritualists believed that on awakening the Kundalini, the latter instantaneously rose to the head and the initiate was automatically united with his Innermost or Internal God, instantly, and converted into Mahatma. How comfortable! How comfortably all these theosophists, Rosicrucians and spiritualists, etc., imagined High Initiation." - Samael Aun Weor, *The Zodiacal Course*

"There are seven bodies of the Being. Each body has its "cerebrospinal" nervous system, its medulla and Kundalini. Each body is a complete organism. There are, therefore, seven bodies, seven medullae and seven Kundalinis. The ascension of each of the seven Kundalinis is slow and difficult. Each canyon or vertebra represents determined occult powers and this is why the conquest of each canyon undergoes terrible tests." - Samael Aun Weor, *The Zodiacal Course*

Logos: (Greek) means Verb or Word. In Greek and Hebrew metaphysics, the unifying principle of the world. The Logos is the manifested deity of every nation and people; the outward expression or the effect of the cause which is ever concealed. (Speech is the "logos" of thought). The Logos has three aspects, known universally as the Trinity or Trimurti. The First Logos is the Father, Brahma. The Second Logos is the Son, Vishnu. The Third Logos is the Holy Spirit, Shiva. One who incarnates the Logos becomes a Logos.

"The Logos is not an individual. The Logos is an army of ineffable beings." - Samael Aun Weor, *Fundamental Notions of Endocrinology and Criminology*

Magic: The word magic is derived from the ancient word "mag" that means priest. Real magic is the work of a priest. A real magician is a priest.

"Magic, according to Novalis, is the art of influencing the inner world consciously." - Samael Aun Weor, *The Mystery of the Golden Blossom*

"When magic is explained as it really is, it seems to make no sense to fanatical people. They prefer to follow their world of illusions." - Samael Aun Weor, *The Revolution of Beelzebub*

Mantra: (Sanskrit, literally "mind protection") A sacred word or sound. The use of sacred words and sounds is universal throughout all religions and mystical traditions, because the root of all creation is in the Great Breath or the Word, the Logos. "In the beginning was the Word..."

Master: Like many terms related to spirituality, this one is grossly misunderstood. Samael Aun Weor wrote while describing the Germanic Edda, "In this Genesis of creation we discover Sexual Alchemy. The Fire fecundated the cold waters of chaos. The masculine principle Alfadur fecundated the feminine principle Niffleheim, dominated by Surtur (the Darkness), to bring forth life. That is how Ymir is born, the father of the giants, the Internal God of every human being, the Master." Therefore, the Master is the Innermost, Atman, the Father.

"The only one who is truly great is the Spirit, the Innermost. We, the intellectual animals, are leaves that the wind tosses about... No student of occultism is a master. True masters are only those who have reached the Fifth Initiation of Major Mysteries. Before the Fifth Initiation nobody is a master." - Samael Aun Weor, *The Perfect Matrimony*

Meditation: "When the esotericist submerges himself into meditation, what he seeks is information." - Samael Aun Weor

"It is urgent to know how to meditate in order to comprehend any psychic aggregate, or in other words, any psychological defect. It is indispensable to know how to work with all our heart and with all our soul, if we want the elimination to occur." - Samael Aun Weor, *The Pistis Sophia Unveiled*

"1. The Gnostic must first attain the ability to stop the course of his thoughts, the capacity to not think. Indeed, only the one who achieves that capacity will hear the Voice of the Silence.

"2. When the Gnostic disciple attains the capacity to not think, then he must learn to concentrate his thoughts on only one thing.

"3. The third step is correct meditation. This brings the first flashes of the new consciousness into the mind.

"4. The fourth step is contemplation, ecstasy or Samadhi. This is the state of Turiya (perfect clairvoyance). - Samael Aun Weor, *The Perfect Matrimony*

Prana: (Sanskrit; Tibetan bindu) Life-principle; the breath of life; energy. The vital breath, which sustains life in a physical body; the primal energy or force, of which other physical forces are manifestations. In the books of Yoga, prana is described as having five modifications, according to its five different functions. These are: prana (the vital energy that controls the breath), apana (the vital energy that carries downward unassimilated food and drink), samana (the vital energy that carries nutrition all over the body), vyama (the vital energy that pervades the entire body), and udana (the vital energy by which the contents of the stomach are ejected through the mouth). The word Prana is also used as a name of the Cosmic Soul, endowed with activity.

Pranayama: (Sanskrit for "restraint (ayama) of prana (energy, life force)") A type of breathing exercise that transforms the life force (sexual energy) of the practitioner.

"Pranayama is a system of sexual transmutation for single persons." - Samael Aun Weor, *The Yellow Book*

Sexual Magic: The word magic is derived from the ancient word magos "one of the members of the learned and priestly class," from O.Pers.

magush, possibly from PIE *magh- "to be able, to have power." [Quoted from Online Etymology Dictionary].

"All of us possess some electrical and magnetic forces within, and, just like a magnet, we exert a force of attraction and repulsion... Between lovers that magnetic force is particularly powerful and its action has a far-reaching effect." - Samael Aun Weor, *The Mystery of the Golden Blossom*

Sexual magic refers to an ancient science that has been known and protected by the purest, most spiritually advanced human beings, whose purpose and goal is the harnessing and perfection of our sexual forces. A more accurate translation of sexual magic would be "sexual priesthood." In ancient times, the priest was always accompanied by a priestess, for they represent the divine forces at the base of all creation: the masculine and feminine, the Yab-Yum, Ying-Yang, Father-Mother: the Elohim. Unfortunately, the term "sexual magic" has been grossly misinterpreted by mistaken persons such as Aleister Crowley, who advocated a host of degenerated practices, all of which belong solely to the lowest and most perverse mentality and lead only to the enslavement of the consciousness, the worship of lust and desire, and the decay of humanity. True, upright, heavenly sexual magic is the natural harnessing of our latent forces, making them active and harmonious with nature and the divine, and which leads to the perfection of the human being.

"People are filled with horror when they hear about sexual magic; however, they are not filled with horror when they give themselves to all kinds of sexual perversion and to all kinds of carnal passion." - Samael Aun Weor, *The Perfect Matrimony*

Solar Bodies: The physical, vital, astral, mental, and causal bodies that are created through the beginning stages of Alchemy/Tantra and that provide a basis for existence in their corresponding levels of nature, just as the physical body does in the physical world. These bodies or vehicles are superior due to being created out of Solar (Christic) Energy, as opposed to the inferior, lunar bodies we receive from nature. Also known as the Wedding Garment (Christianity), the Merkabah (Kabbalah), To Soma Heliakon (Greek), and Sahu (Egyptian).

"All the Masters of the White Lodge, the Angels, Archangels, Thrones, Seraphim, Virtues, etc., etc., etc. are garbed with the Solar Bodies. Only those who have Solar Bodies have the Being incarnated. Only someone who possesses the Being is an authentic Human Being." - Samael Aun Weor, *The Esoteric Treatise of Hermetic Astrology*

Tattva: (Sanskrit) "truth, fundamental principle." A reference to the essential nature of a given thing. Tattvas are the elemental forces of nature. There are numerous systems presenting varying tattvas as fundamental principles of nature. Gnosticism utilizes a primary system of five: akash (which is the elemental force of the ether), tejas (fire), vayu (air), apas (water) and prittvi (earth). Two higher tattvas are also important: adi and samadhi.

White Brotherhood: That ancient collection of pure souls who maintain the highest and most sacred of sciences: White Magic or White Tantra. It is called white due to its purity and cleanliness. This "brotherhood" or "lodge" includes human beings of the highest order from every race, culture, creed and religion, and of both sexes.

Index

About the Author

His name is Hebrew סמאל און ואור, and is pronounced "sam-ayel on vay-or." You may not have heard of him, but Samael Aun Weor changed the world.

In 1950, in his first two books, he became the first person to reveal the esoteric secret hidden in all the world's great religions, and for that, accused of "healing the ill," he was put in prison. Nevertheless, he did not stop. Between 1950 and 1977 – merely twenty-seven years – not only did Samael Aun Weor write over sixty books on the most difficult subjects in the world, such as consciousness, kabbalah, physics, tantra, meditation, etc., in which he deftly exposed the singular root of all knowledge — which he called Gnosis — he simultaneously inspired millions of people across the entire span of Latin America: stretching across twenty countries and an area of more than 21,000,000 kilometers, founding schools everywhere, even in places without electricity or post offices.

During those twenty-seven years, he experienced all the extremes that humanity could give him, from adoration to death threats, and in spite of the enormous popularity of his books and lectures, he renounced an income, refused recognitions, walked away from accolades, and consistently turned away those who would worship him. He held as friends both presidents and peasants, and yet remained a mystery to all.

When one reflects on the effort and will it requires to perform even day to day tasks, it is astonishing to consider the herculean efforts required to accomplish what he did in such a short time. But, there is a reason: he was a man who knew who he was, and what he had to do. A true example of compassion and selfless service, Samael Aun Weor dedicated the whole of his life to freely helping anyone and everyone find the path out of suffering. His mission was to show all of humanity the universal source of all spiritual traditions, which he did not only through his writings and lectures, but also through his actions. He said,

"I do not want to receive visitors. Unquestionably, I am nothing more than a postman, a courier, a man that delivers a message... It would be the breaking point of silliness for you to come from your country to the capital city of Mexico with the only purpose of visiting a vulgar postman, an employee that delivered you a letter in the past... Why would you waste your money for that? Why would you visit a simple courier, a miserable postman? It is better for you to study the message, the written teachings delivered in the books...

"I have not come to form any sect, or one more belief, nor am I interested in the schools of today, or the particular beliefs of anyone! ...

"We are not interested in anyone's money, nor are we interested in monthly fees, or temples made out of brick, cement or clay, because we are conscious visitors in the cathedral of the soul and we know that wisdom is of the soul.

"Flattery tires us, praise should only belong to our Father (who is in secret and watches over us minutely).

"We are not in search of followers; all we want is for each person to follow his or her self— their own internal master, their sacred Innermost—because he is the only one who can save and glorify us.

"I do not follow anyone, therefore no one should follow me...

"We do not want any more comedies, pretenses, false mysticism, or false schools. What we want now are living realities; we want to prepare ourselves to see, hear, and touch the reality of those truths..." —Samael Aun Weor